RESETTING
THE CLOCK

RESETTING THE CLOCK

5 Anti-Aging Hormones That Are Revolutionizing the Quality and Length of Life

ELMER CRANTON, M.D., AND WILLIAM FRYER

M. Evans and Company, Inc.
New York

DISCLAIMER

The ideas and advice in the book are based upon the experience and training of the author and the scientific information currently available. The suggestions in this book are definitely not meant to be a substitute for careful medical evaluation and treatment by a qualified, licensed health professional. The author and publisher do not recommend changing medication or adding hormones without consulting your personal physician. They specifically disclaim any liability arising directly or indirectly from the use of this book.

M. Evans and Company, Inc.
216 East 49th Street
New York, New York 10017

Library of Congress Cataloging-in-Publication Data

Cranton, Elmer M.
    Resetting the clock : 5 anti-aging hormones that are revolutionizing the quality and length of life / Elmer Cranton and William Fryer.
        p.   cm.
    Includes bibliographical references and index.
    ISBN 0-87131-801-6 (cloth)
    1. Longevity.   2. Aging—Hormone therapy.   I. Fryer, William, 1949-   . II. Title.
    RA776.75.C7   1996   96-23750
    612.6'8—dc20   CIP

Design and formatting by Bernard Schleifer

Manufactured in the United States of America

9   8   7   6   5   4   3   2

Contents

Preface

THIS BOOK IS BASED ON INTERVIEWS WITH HUNDREDS OF SCIEN-
tists and on the case histories of hundreds of patients. The
hormone revolution that is now under way is irreversible
and astonishing. We wrote this book out of a conviction
that the public at large has a right to know the kinds of
choices they will soon be offered in controlling their own
longevity. There are risks as well as advantages in hor-
monally changing the course of human aging, but it seems
to us that only a fair evaluation of the evidence will equip
people to weigh the one against the other.

The human race has had a long experience with aging.
If the type of aging we are going to experience is now going
to change forever—and the authors of this book believe it
certainly is—then we had best ask ourselves as soon as
possible what we are going to achieve, why we want to get
there, how much we are willing to pay for a longer ride, and
what the ultimate destiny of a human race that does not
peter out and die at seventy-five or eighty is going to be.

All these questions and more are part of the substance
of this book. We could not have written it without the coop-
eration of many people, men and women, laypersons and
scientists, patients and doctors, young and old. Thanks to
every one of them. May they live abundantly protected by

their hormones and with the fullest possible measure of youth's vigor for a hundred years or more.

It is only fair and prudent to add that nothing in this book is intended to provide individual medical advice for individual people. You should choose your own health care and your own path to a longer life with the aid of a competent and caring physician.

ELMER CRANTON, M.D.
WILLIAM FRYER

PART I

Hormones Change Everything

CHAPTER ONE

The Promise of Longevity

"Aging and death do seem to be what Nature has planned for us. But what if we have other plans?"

—BERNARD STREHLER, gerontologist

LIFE ENDS. THIS WE KNOW. IF I COULD PROMISE YOU IMMORTALITY, I'd do so right now, but I'm a mere mortal, a doctor, a scientist, a healer. Not, alas, a representative of the deity. I can't in all honesty say that I'm going to show you how to live forever. But to give you some idea of what I can show you, let me turn the tables and ask you a few simple questions.

How would you like to stay healthy far into old age? Not simply breathing but retaining vitality and enthusiasm, enough of both to make life well worth living. And what, for you personally, is the numerical definition of old age? Perhaps your expectations of its limits are a mite on the conservative side. Would you like a longer life? Suppose you were offered a bit extra—ten years, twenty years longer than your family history would lead you to expect. Imagine for a moment that the quality of that added life turns out to be far closer to what you enjoyed at thirty than to what you fear to experience at eighty. Are these impossible fantasies?

They won't seem to be once you've read these pages. I'm going to devote the next sixteen chapters to telling you about the rise of the pro-longevity hormones—perhaps the most startling series of developments medicine has seen in decades. Indeed, perhaps the most genuinely unusual transformations the art and science of health care has ever undergone. A staggering assault on aging—and one that few people anticipated.

I certainly didn't. As little as five years ago, I had no expectation that replacement of the age-depleted hormones in the human body would allow people to live a substantially longer and healthier life. Probably not one doctor in a thousand had even heard a rumor when this decade began, and even today only a small minority of physicians is well informed about the hormones (with the exception of the sex hormones) that this book will be discussing.

Consequently, the subject matter of *Resetting the Clock* is markedly different from what you'll find in most current medical books proposing to tell you how to stop aging. Good books, many of them, and I imagine that many of you are already doing what they advise. You've been told that a prudent lifestyle is the ticket to long life. It's good advice, as far as it goes. I'm certainly proud that for more than two decades now I've been encouraging my patients to eat well, exercise, and take nutritional supplements.

Such simple steps frequently change aging lives so effectively that instead of lurching into their sixties ready for their first heart attack and rightly depressed about their physical future, men and women carry on with fairly good energy until they're eighty-five or ninety. How wonderful compared to the alternatives!

But not in any way exceptional. I'll offer a few chapters of recommendations along those lines in Part II, but useful as I've tried to make them, they are in no way the main burden of this book.

Instead, I have a message for you which is simply this: a veritable hormone revolution has rewritten the rule book for human aging. The process of getting older as the human race has known it for thousands of years is about to be—is actually in the process of being—changed utterly. The longer and conspicuously healthier life that I'm proposing for anyone who will reach out and take it will be up around 100, 110, or 120. Those are the outer limits of longevity right now. Only about one out of every fifty human beings now makes it to the century mark. A woman in Arles, France, recently clocked in at 121 and became the oldest human being for whom reliable records exist. She is an oddity, a gerontological anomaly right now. In a few more decades, believe me, she isn't going to seem so odd.

TESTING THE WATERS

In a small way, the hormone revolution has already begun. The very first of the pro-longevity hormones began surging into prominence more than thirty years ago. That was estrogen.

In the 1990s more than fifty million American women will reach menopause, and at least 20 percent of them will take sex hormones to ease the passage. A very large percentage of these hormonal adventurers will then go on to take them for life.

This mass supplementation with the female sex hormones is far more revolutionary than people realize. Although the pro-longevity effects of estrogen and progesterone are quite limited compared to some of the other hormones we'll be discussing, the principle is the same. People are putting back into their bodies what the aging process has taken out. And, for the most part, they're finding that they like it.

The results are worth cheering about. Millions of women have been on sex hormone replacement therapy for decades. Using present day methods of administration, the likelihood of increased cancer risk has been shown to be extremely small, and virtually every sizable study of post-menopausal women has proven that women who take hormones live longer and are generally far healthier than women who don't. Good news for the human race.

But although nearly every bit of new scientific information indicates that even better news is on the way for all of us, male and female alike, the subject matter of this book remains controversial to its core. DHEA, human growth hormone, testosterone, melatonin—to name the most significant of the substances I'll be telling you about—are not yet prescribed by most physicians. They are being vigorously studied and hotly debated in academic circles. Because the immense attractiveness of the effects they produce is supported by only five to ten years of experimental studies on humans, many conservative medical authorities see them as a potentially reckless alteration of the normal practice of both medicine and aging.

I don't agree with that, and I would certainly be willing to argue my case—indeed, I'm about to—but very probably the whole controversy is going to be taken right out of our hands. The American public will do it. I know my countrymen well enough to predict they won't be satisfied with one sip from the fountain of youth.

Estrogen is a mere beginning. It, too, sprang into widespread use without extensive preliminary testing, largely because the terrifying effects of osteoporosis on aging women virtually mandated its use in spite of considerable resistance from a cautious medical world. Now, as the chapters ahead will show you, the pro-longevity hormones promise a reprieve of sentence for the most terrifying health hazard of all—aging itself. And the most extraordinary thing about these hormones is that they're not *extraordinary*—they're utterly natural. They're the very substances that our bodies secreted abundantly when we were young. And now we know that those substances have youth in them.

We are the carriers of our own youth. It flows within us, magical and rich. Then, as age dries us up, we become the hollowed-out sticks, the mere stiff and painfully uninvigorated caricatures of what we were. Of course, we have never had options in these matters. Age did with us what it would. Our creaky joints and flaccid muscles, our sadly depleted sex drive, our tired days and unsettled nights were our destiny. At least until now.

Point of Departure

In 1990 a team of researchers at the University of Wisconsin led by Dr. Daniel Rudman published a revolutionizing paper in the *New England Journal of Medicine*. Its simple title: "Effects of Human Growth Hormone in Men Over 60 Years Old."[1]

What should growth hormone have to do with men over sixty? Growth hormone is critical for the growth of children and falls steadily once adulthood is reached. Few doctors had ever considered giving it to grown-ups. But when the twenty-one healthy elderly men in Dr. Rudman's study were given it, they quite literally grew. They grew muscle, they grew a thicker and healthier skin, they grew bone density. Inevitably something was lost: fat. If these men were like others who have been studied since, they probably also grew larger and more durable livers, kidneys, and spleens, for our organs shrink, too, as we grow old.

In many respects, Rudman's men grew young. After six months of treatment, many of them looked ten to fifteen years younger than when they started.

Reported in the newspapers then, but largely forgotten since, this was one of the first drumbeats of the hormone revolution.

What's Nature; What's Age?

What's aging? Why does it occur? Clearly nature has worked out a system of planned obsolescence for all of us. Just as clearly most of us intend to thwart nature's designs for as long as we're able.

Many theories have been hatched in an attempt to explain our decline. Some scientists believe that every time cells divide, the copying mechanism introduces new errors in our DNA—that's the "worn template" theory. Others believe that our bodies are gradually poisoned by an accumulation of chemical toxins that they can no longer effectively excrete. Long-term failure of the immune system is a hypothesis that has attracted many supporters; certainly, as we grow older, there is a progressive decline in the immune system's ability to detect and destroy infections and developing cancers.

All of these theories may well form part of a complex whole. It certainly seems true that our bodies are in some larger sense organized for decline. Many gerontologists have theorized the existence of an "aging clock," an orderly process whose command center or centers we have not yet identified but from which, nevertheless, a message goes to our various organs and glands that says: Time's up! There's a mechanism inside each of our cells, which I'll be explaining in the very last chapter, that clearly has a major role to play in clocking our demise.

But, when all our theories have been considered, there is certainly no doubt that much of the aging we so visibly notice is tied to the slowing of hormonal systems that do not seem to have been significantly damaged by toxins or misbehaving cells. They simply are not producing what they used to produce. An invisible timer has slowed their pace. Men and women who take care of themselves, who are relatively unstressed, well exercised, intelligently nourished, and entirely healthy, nonetheless—once they pass their youthful prime—find themselves secreting progressively smaller amounts of the hormones that are essential to life.

Why this occurs is uncertain. The fact that it occurs is absolutely as well documented as the rising of the sun is well observed. Our vital fluids, so to speak, are draining away. If you were ghoulishly inclined, you might say that you were being vampirized by your own body.

At the present time, this is the most interesting aspect of aging because we can do something about it. The hormones that keep us young are now readily replaceable.

What are these hormones? Let me name them briefly. The most important ones, according to our present knowledge, are:

- *Human Growth Hormone (HGH)*—always known to be vital in childhood, this is now recognized as a major player in the repair and upkeep of the adult body and has such startling effects in older people that it alone may significantly extend longevity and vastly improve quality of life.

- *DHEA (dehydroepiandrosterone)*—this, our chief adrenal hormone, has many mysterious roles and functions in the body. If we now recognize its importance, it is largely because we observe the extraordinary effects that supplementation with it can produce.

- *Melatonin*—the major product of our brain's pineal gland, melatonin certainly ensures a good night's sleep, but, more importantly, it may control the body's aging clock.

- **Estrogen and progesterone**—the female body does not respond favorably to the sudden and almost total deprivation of its sex hormones at menopause. Postmenopausal women who replace them know how significantly vitalizing estrogen and progesterone can be, statisticians know that women who take them live longer, and someday all women may know what a sacrifice they are making if they avoid them.

- **Testosterone**—the male hormone has become some men's secret weapon against aging. Will it go mainstream, as estrogen has done? We are on the verge of such a breakthrough.

MIRROR, MIRROR ON THE WALL, HOW DO MY HORMONES FALL?

You started life with ample supplies of some of these vital substances. When you reached puberty, the sex hormones kicked in, and things really changed. At the same time, the hormones that directly promote growth, energy, and strength began surging to new heights. From your early teens to your mid-twenties, you had a physical force and dynamism that probably astonishes you when you look back upon it. And then—very slowly, at first—this energy, the strength to move mountains, diminished. By the time most of us are forty, we realize we're no longer quite so young. By the time we're fifty, "middle-aged"—a stuffy, unexciting expression if ever there was one—seems like our inevitable self-description. Soon, as the years pass, there's no way to escape it—we're not young anymore, we can't climb mountains and we probably don't want to.

But I'd like you to remember that this inevitable, time-related decline in hormonal vitality seems to affect some individuals differently. It's not that they don't have an aging clock, but it's set on a different time.

If you think about it, you'll realize that there have always been people who by some accident of natural endowment seem to temporarily negate the hard-headed certainties of aging. Indeed, in any century, there are men and women who amaze their contemporaries by what they do in old age. Winston Churchill was running the affairs of embattled wartime England in his seventies, and, then, in his next five years of enforced retirement, wrote a massive six-volume history of the Second World War. Giuseppe Verdi composed two of his greatest operas in his early eighties. Grandma Moses was painting pictures throughout her eighties, and Picasso was going strong until almost ninety. But this sort of extended vigorous life is not confined to the exceptionally talented. Humbler folk, like you and me, are busy even as I write, managing their businesses, farming their acres, or carrying on their medical practices in their eighties or nineties. Unusual, yes, but definitely common enough that many of us have met one or two examples.

It is a very safe bet that each of these individuals had—by some accident of genetic endowment—the capacity to retain relatively high levels of essential hormones into old age. Without those hormones, all the character and determination in the world would not have been enough to keep them functioning at a high level in the home stretch. Very simply, the wheels don't turn without gas in the tank.

But even these lucky people weren't functioning the way they did when they were young. What if, in addition to their relatively bountiful natural endowments, they had been taking supplemental doses of hormones so that their levels of growth hormone, DHEA, melatonin, and the major sex hormones had been raised to what they had when young?

The experiences of my patients and the evidence of carefully conducted scientific studies reported in the med-

ical journals of the world strongly suggest that they would
have been even more vital and energetic than they were.
And there is certainly reason to think many of them would
have lived longer.

The experiences of experimental animals lucky enough
to have received hormone replacement therapy is that life
spans can be extended by as much as 30 percent. We don't
know if we can achieve an increase in longevity that great
in humans, because no one has been supplemented with
the major hormones for a long enough period to show such
increases. The whole medical world—at least that part of it
whose interest is centered on gerontology, the science of
aging—is watching and waiting.

Changing Nature?

But is this the path we wish to follow? It certainly must be
clear to you by now that I'm proposing nothing less than a
complete reversal of the body's natural process of hormonal
decline. As you get older, melatonin, human growth hormone, DHEA, estrogen, and testosterone will go down radically and, until the development of hormone replacement
therapy, irreversibly. As you'll see in the next few chapters,
there's nothing subtle about these falls. When it comes to
hormones, a normal seventy-year-old is making do with
short rations; a normal ninety-year-old is alarmingly close
to an empty tank.

This hormone drop is part of nature's plan. We see it in
animals just as reliably as in humans. Dare we interfere
with the planned depletion of the hormonal reservoir?

I honestly don't see how we could be true to ourselves if
we didn't. First of all, let me note that before the twentieth
century, a clear majority of human beings never got old
enough to be adversely affected by a decline in hormone
levels. As late as 1890, the average life expectancy was

around forty-five years. A whole lot's changed since then, including better water supplies, vastly improved sanitation, less crowded living conditions, more adequate housing, central heating, and a host of medical breakthroughs.

If it's unnatural to interfere with planned hormonal obsolescence as we age, then I'd certainly like to know how that unnatural interference differs from all the other equally unnatural things we've been doing in medicine since 1900. In this century we declared war on microbes by developing vaccines and inventing antibiotics. Infectious and parasitic diseases used to kill the largest portion of men and women. Not anymore. In the last forty years surgery got its turn. Amazing creative solutions to intractable medical dilemmas. In your wildest dreams, can you imagine anything more unnatural than organ transplants?

I don't think it makes sense to belabor this point. It's quite clear God wouldn't have given us the abilities we possess if we weren't supposed to use them. If there's anything that's really and truly natural to us it's the compulsion to forge the best possible life for ourselves. No question that for most people that will include the longest and healthiest span of years on this earth that human ingenuity—a natural endowment, if ever there was one—can devise.

The pro-longevity hormones are the great transformers. What vaccinations and antibiotics were to the twentieth century, they will be to the twenty-first. Get out your timepieces, folks, we're about to reset the clock.

WILL THIS BE YOU?

How much can the pro-longevity hormones do for one? Let me offer an example.

There is a man in Florida named Carl Everett. He's a very interesting human being. Carl is a successful stockbroker. He works full time at it and has for many years. In his youth, Carl was a navy pilot flying from aircraft carriers. He's married now, settled down and well satisfied with life.

Carl's always been a physically active person, and his daily regimen includes a three-and-a-half-mile run along the beach. He also belongs to a scuba diving club. He just got back from diving in the Red Sea, and last year he went diving off Honduras in the Caribbean and explored some of the underwater caves on that Central American country's coast. Carl generally dives three or four times a month, often going as deep as one to two hundred feet. Those who know something about diving will tell you that the physical strain of reaching such depths is considerable. Carl Everett, however, keeps up with his scuba diving comrades without difficulty.

Which is intriguing, because Carl is seventy-five years old, and none of the men he dives with is over fifty. Carl has been taking injections of human growth hormone for the past twelve years and swallowing a daily dose of the adrenal hormone DHEA for the past six.

I sometimes think Carl Everett may be the face of the future.

CHAPTER TWO

Visiting the Hormone Kingdom: Your Glands and You

MANY OF MY READERS WILL HAVE A ONE-SIDED AND SOMEWHAT negative preconceived notion about "hormones." Aren't they something that makes teenagers wild and sexually crazed, that makes women with PMS miserable and cranky, that has some connection with getting fat, feeling depressed, and developing acne? Won't hormones cause cancer?

Well, there's a little bit of truth in all of those fears. Anything as potent as hormones has the potential to be harmful, if not used properly. Hormones must be harmonized; they must be kept in perfect balance, just like the instruments in a symphony orchestra. As we age, that balance is interrupted by a disproportionate decline in some of the more essential hormones, creating an imbalance and discord in our bodies. The resulting symptoms are often considered to be inevitable accompaniments of aging.

Our goal is to restore a harmonizing balance in a very natural and healthy way. If hormones are not balanced, and if some are given in excess relative to others, adverse side effects will occur. Anything that has a major role to play in the body can have a negative role to play as well if misused.

Hormones can be very potent, and even tiny amounts can have major effects. Adrenaline, for example, is secreted in such minute amounts that the concentration necessary to produce a fight-or-flight reaction is equivalent to one drop in a railroad tank car.

Endocrine glands secrete hormones directly into your bloodstream. From there, they get carried to other organs and to tissues throughout your body. All the pro-longevity hormones discussed in this book are endocrine hormones. So we'd better inspect the glands from which they originate.

Suppose you're walking down Main Street when a tiger steps out from between two parked cars, opens its large, toothy mouth and, fixing that special look on you that tigers always reserve for tasty morsels, roars hungrily. Your heart begins to pound very fast, you start to move away, and as soon as you're within sprinting distance of a solid door, you cover the ground in record time, open the door, and slam it shut just an instant before six hundred pounds of big cat arrives on the other side, late for lunch. You notice that you're shaking badly. That was an adrenaline surge! Adrenaline, which originates in the central core of the adrenal glands, is the fight-or-flight hormone released into the bloodstream in response to stress.

Or, more realistically, let's say it's May, the time when young people's hearts turn to romance, and you're a young man. You're walking down Main Street when suddenly you see that special young lady walking toward you, as ravishing as ever, charmingly costumed, and smiling your way. Your heart begins to beat harder, your whole body begins to tingle, and the combination of sensations, emotions, and anticipations you're experiencing is fairly inde-scribable. The suggestion that romance is nothing more than hormones is one I'd never dream of making, but I'm sure there's testosterone involved in this equation somewhere. Testosterone is the male sex hormone pro-duced primarily in the testicles but also, to a lesser extent, in the adrenals.

We're talking endocrinology, and when I tell you that this extraordinary team of hormones secreted by the endocrine glands not only powers your flight-or-fight mech-anism and underlies your sex drive but also permits you to grow, allows you to fight infection and heal injury, controls your inner heating apparatus, permits and encourages a good night's sleep, balances the levels of minerals in your body, and adjusts the burning of fuel for energy—then I think you'll understand that deploying the proper quanti-ties of these natural substances daily is every bit as crucial to your continued existence as breathing air.

Moreover, it's now known that the endocrine glands are crucially involved in the timing mechanism of your aging clock. We don't just wear out as we get older, we are phased out. There is a precise, hidden pattern of messages com-municating from our glands to the rest of our bodies that corresponds to how far we've come and how far we still have to go. Naturally, accident or illness—perhaps self-inflicted due to our lifestyles—can terminate our time on this planet long before our biological clocks would other-wise have run down. But even if we live with wonderful prudence, the clock is ticking.

Can it be slowed? Can the hands of the clock be turned back? We're not certain, but our present knowledge indi-cates that the hormonal approach offers us the best chance yet for performing such delicate clockwork alterations. Scientists have succeeded in giving mice life spans that are 30 percent greater than the normal maximum for that species. In my view, that's adjusting the biological clock.

One of the most effective methods used has been endocrine supplementation. Hormone secretion decreases at a predictable rate with age in humans as well as mice. By merely restoring levels to those present in healthy young adulthood, many of the adverse accompaniments of old age can, at least partially, be reversed and forestalled in the future.

Before we consider this novel method for extending your life span and for improving the quality of your more mature years, let's look at the endocrine system gland by gland.

FROM THE BOTTOM UP

We'll start our tour with the gonads—the woman's ovaries and the man's testes. These are the endocrine system's chief production plants for the sex hormones.

We're all familiar with the physical results of the sex hormones—the curves, the breast development, the softer skin of women; the larger muscles, the deeper voice, the relative hairiness of men. Certainly the functional differences in anatomy and the specialization of reproductive function are sufficiently obvious, too. Though many hormones combine in the production of these delightful variations, the two dominant stimulators are testosterone in men and estrogen in women.

That's not the end of the effective action undertaken by these potent anabolic steroids—which is, of course, what the sex hormones are. Anabolic means that they stimulate growth and healing of tissues. These hormones support protein synthesis, bone structure, skin tone, muscle strength, the health and functioning of neural networks in the brain, and many other aspects of strength and vitality. It is not surprising that the sex hormones have such powerful effects. Youthfulness is strongly associated with physical vigor as well as sexual vitality. Nothing more vividly indicates that we're still young, still participants in the game of life, than our sexual urges.

It's only logical to ask whether, by reversing an age-related decline in the sex hormones, we can reverse other aspects of aging as well. And, certainly, the answer appears to be a qualified yes. The last twenty years have fully demonstrated the powerfully vitalizing effects of estrogen supplementation on postmenopausal women; there are some indications that the next twenty will show somewhat similar effects in males who use testosterone supplementally. In the case of men, however, a fundamental difference (which we'll explore in Chapter Ten) is that the degree to which male testosterone levels decline with age is far less predictable.

Moving slightly upward in the body we reach the uterus in women and the prostate gland in men. They are, of course, closely related to the sex organs, part of the whole apparatus of reproduction. During pregnancy the uterus manufactures massive quantities of progesterone in order to promote normal functioning of the placenta, the link between the blood supply of the mother and the baby.

The prostate gland—source of so much male discomfort in the second half of life—produces various constituents of seminal fluid and also contains a tiny vestigial uterus that never develops further in men. Unfortunately, in the anti-aging scheme of things, the prostate's function is often a negative one; it's the prime male site for cancer. And it often tends to enlarge with age, causing obstruction to the flow of urine from the bladder.

The Tour Continues

The next endocrine gland that we reach in our journey toward the brain is the pancreas, the source of your body's insulin. In healthy people, the pancreas will function efficiently until the end of life, but in people with diabetes there is (depending on the type of diabetes) either a shortage of insulin or a resistance in the body to insulin's effects. Insulin does not really have a place as a pro-longevity hormone. Without it you would simply die. Fortunately, since 1922 it has been possible to provide it by injection to successfully treat diabetes.

Insulin is released whenever we eat carbohydrates such as starches or sugar. It functions to facilitate the transport of blood sugar (glucose) into our cells for fuel. Glucose is stored in the liver and muscles as a complex carbohydrate called glycogen. If insulin is not doing its job properly, then the excess glucose is more easily converted to fat and the breakdown of fat for energy is also impaired. On the other hand, if insulin takes too much glucose out of the blood stream (hypoglycemia), we feel weak and tired and counterregulatory hormones (largely created by the adrenal glands) are released to convert glycogen and/or fat back into glucose, the body's main source of energy.

It's quite typical for the body to use insulin less efficiently as we get older, but careful diet and exercise can minimize that problem.

Twin Powerhouses

Traveling upward we pass the kidneys and find, at the top of each of them, two little but spectacularly potent glands called the adrenals. In their center (the medullas), the adrenal glands produce adrenaline, the hormone that so spectacularly jump-starts our emergency action system. Adrenaline ignites a high speed burn-off of the starch called glycogen that insulin stores in our muscles and livers. This causes an almost instantaneous rise in blood levels of glucose, fueling the flood of energy that we need for action. Adrenaline also speeds the heartbeat and the breathing rate.

On the outer layer or cortex of the adrenals, one of the body's major hormones, DHEA (dehydroepiandrosterone), is manufactured from cholesterol, and from DHEA the body makes a wide spectrum of other steroid hormones, including aldosterone, which preserves minerals in the body, and cortisone, which controls immune responses and also affects energy and mineral metabolism.

DHEA is also the raw material from which the repro- ductive organs make the sex hormones, and thus it is now justifiably regarded as one of the most important hormones in the human body. It is significant, therefore, that DHEA declines steadily and predictably with age. When you're in your twenties, your cup is filled to overflowing with DHEA. After that, the long slide starts.

DHEA is sensitive to the immediate conditions of your physical and mental life. Illness depletes it, as does severe stress of any kind.

A Gland That Shrivels

The next hormone-producing center is in the chest behind the heart and is called the thymus gland. The thymus is one of the major organs of the immune system—indeed, in childhood, it's absolutely essential to developing an immune system in the first place. Its principal task is the creation of T lymphocytes, the specialized cells (killer cells) that find helper cell lymphocytes and eliminate bacteria, viruses, and foreign matter from the body. In late childhood the thymus is the size of a plum, but at puberty it begins to shrink. By the time we reach old age, it's the size of a small raisin and relatively inactive. It's interesting that, statisti- cally, a human being is least likely to die at the age of twelve, when his or her thymus is in full flower. Although some of the functions of the thymus actually get transferred from the thymus to other areas—such as the lymph nodes and bone marrow—as we get older, so that we can continue to make lymphocytes, there's still good reason for thinking that the steady shrinking of the thymus is bad news and heralds the eventual decline and fall of our immune system.

The good news is that three of the pro-longevity hormones I'll be telling you about—DHEA, melatonin, and growth hormone—can slow or, in some experiments, actually reverse the shrinkage of the thymus. By so doing, they slow, perhaps even halt, the decline of immunity with age. And a body that can defend itself against illness is a body that is far more likely to live into a second century.

In Charge of the Furnace

The next stopping point on our endocrine tour of the body is the thyroid, a butterfly-shaped gland about two inches wide and weighing about an ounce, which is located just beneath the voice box at the front of the throat. This remarkable little organ regulates our metabolism. That is to say, it controls the production of energy in our cells. When the fuel from food and stored fat is combined with oxygen in our cells, chemical energy is produced. That is what powers movement, body heat, cellular activity, muscular activity, growth, healing, circulation, brain function, and every other function necessary for life. We'll talk about the thyroid—its proper functioning, its occasional disorders—in Appendix One.

Thyroid hormone sometimes diminishes unduly with age, a condition called hypothyroidism. Less often, the thyroid becomes overactive and produces excessive thyroid hormone. The effects of either state can be quite damaging to one's health. A person with insufficient levels of thyroid hormone (hypothyroidism) will feel sluggish and cold, will gain weight, and will experience a slowdown in most of the body's vital functions. Overproduction of thyroid hormone (hyperthyroidism) causes fatigue, anxiety, tremulousness, sweating, weight loss, and sometimes heart failure.

Fortunately, modern medicine is quite capable of normalizing thyroid production or supplementing inadequacies as needed. More problematic is diagnosing the difficulty to start with. Controversy swirls around the most effective methods of determining thyroid malfunction. I'll be talking about these methods at some length. A malfunctioning thyroid is definitely not conducive to good health and longevity.

And Now for the Command Centers

The thyroid gland's production of hormone is controlled by another hormone, TSH (thyroid-stimulating hormone), which is itself a product of the pituitary gland. Many a medical writer before me has somewhat colorfully termed the pituitary the body's "master gland." I agree with that description. Once we arrive at the pituitary, we truly have reached a higher order of endocrine gland.

With a few exceptions, such as growth hormone, the pituitary does not produce the hormones that do the heavy labor of regulating physical processes. Instead, it produces hormones to stimulate the other endocrine glands to produce their hormones. Thus by means of a hormone called ACTH (adrenal cortical stimulating hormone), the pituitary governs the output of specific adrenal cortical hormones by the adrenal gland. In a similar fashion, it directs the production of the sex hormones through pituitary-controlling hormones called gonadotrophins (trophic means "to stimulate the growth of").

The advantages of such a system are plain. The pituitary is the guardian of a balanced production of endocrine chemicals. It functions much like the thermostat in your home to regulate heating or cooling systems. If the body begins to produce too much estrogen or testosterone, too much thyroid hormone, or too much cortisone, then the pituitary lowers its output of stimulating hormones, and endocrine production in the lower glands declines. If hormone levels are too low, then the chemical message causes the "thermostat" to be turned up. In medical language, this is called a feedback system, and, if you are healthy, it works beautifully.

The pituitary is a small organ at the base of the brain, hidden and protected in the middle of the head. It weighs less than a gram (one-fortieth of an ounce) and is connected by a thin stalk to the hypothalamus, which is the lowermost part of the brain itself. Perhaps the hypothalamus, as part of the brain, should be called the master gland! These two glands function in such close interconnection that they can hardly be thought of apart. The hypothalamus has sensors that detect circulating blood levels of the many specific hormones that the pituitary controls. In response to the information, it sends chemical messengers to the pituitary to turn production by the lower endocrine centers up or down as needed.

The hypothalamus really is the body's thermostat—and quite literally so in matters of temperature. We only function efficiently when our temperature is within a degree or so of the ideal 98.6 degrees Fahrenheit, which is the conventional number quoted in the textbooks. Each of us may vary from that slightly. But if our temperature is more than one degree above or below our personal ideal, we begin to experience symptoms of malfunction. The hypothalamus has a whole range of techniques for bringing us back to normal, starting with the most obvious: shivering to heat us when we're cold and perspiring to cool us when we're hot.

More delicately, the hypothalamus signals the pituitary to signal the thyroid that something's amiss. And the thyroid, through its control of energy release with thyroid hormone, definitely has the capacity to do something about it.

Before we go on to the last endocrine gland, the pineal, we must mention that the pituitary has another function and releases another hormone that has a major function throughout the body all on its own—human growth hormone (HGH). It is rather ironic that this is the substance that more obviously than any other seems capable of altering human aging. Until just a few years ago, HGH was considered a profoundly uninteresting and nearly unnecessary hormone once we reached adulthood. Perhaps the name was part of the confusion. Clearly needed for the growth of children, what was the point of a "growth" hormone once we had achieved our full growth? We now know that HGH is vitally necessary all through life; it's your body's all-purpose repair and maintenance hormone.

The source of our education is people who lost their pituitaries or who, for some congenital reason, are unable to produce growth hormone. When that happens in childhood, growth virtually comes to a halt. Before growth hormone became available, such children matured as dwarfs, the so-called "Tiny Tim" syndrome. In the 1970s, growth hormone extracted from the pituitaries of human cadavers became available in minute quantities and was used exclusively for the clinical treatment of children with the most severe growth deficiencies. Then in 1985, genetic engineering produced growth hormone from recombinant DNA, and the potential supply of the hormone became limitless. Without that development, it's quite likely we wouldn't have felt inspired to write this book, for it now appears that HGH is the most powerful pro-longevity hormone so far uncovered.

You see, since 1985 it has become clear that, important as growth hormone is to children, it is equally important to adults, but in a different way. The children who grew to normal size with the aid of supplemental HGH have found after they were taken off the hormone that being a growth-hormone-deprived adult is also full of problems. Muscle strength and energy are low. Cell regrowth, repair of injuries, and upkeep of major organs declines. Adults who lose their pituitaries due to surgery or accident almost immediately suffer these same problems, even if they are receiving supplements of all the other hormones for which the pituitary is responsible. This is starting to change for those who are lucky enough to have physicians who can obtain and will prescribe HGH for them. In Chapter Three we'll look at some of the extraordinary transformations— virtual rebirths of vitality—that growth-hormone-deficient adults have enjoyed once their deficiency is corrected. But remember, HGH declines with age in virtually everyone.

The significance of all this for you and me is that, once we reach old age, we are by definition "growth-hormone-deficient adults!"

Your Body's Clock?

Finally we come to the pineal, which has been and to some extent still is the body's mystery gland. As far as we know, the pineal has only one function: to produce the hormone melatonin. A spate of books published during the last year, combined with massive media coverage, has insured that very few readers will be unaware that melatonin is supposed to be good for you. I also believe that it is good for you, and it will be discussed at length in Chapters Seven and Eight. What we don't know for sure is whether the pineal, through its release of melatonin, is also important in actually regulating the body's rate of aging. There is interesting and suggestive evidence from animal studies indicating it just might have that function.

THE WHOLE PICTURE

Looking at the glands we've described above, you will see a very elegant, complex, and interrelated system that controls the most vital parts of our physical and mental functioning. The so-called vegetative functions such as digesting, breathing, and blood circulation tend to be more autonomous, but even those rely on a proper balance of hormones, to some extent. Most of our most important bodily functions are regulated by our endocrine hormones without our even thinking about it.

Need to burn fuel for heat and energy? Your thyroid will conscientiously command the rate of production, acting in response to guidance from the hypothalamus and the pituitary. Although thyroid problems are not uncommon, for many of us they will never occur.

Must dodge danger or hasten to rescue a loved one? Your adrenals will release adrenaline quicker than a flash. And so on, down the whole list of important functions we've been considering.

Now, what goes wrong as we get older? Not everything, happily. We still make adrenaline when in some great crisis it's required. If we're not afflicted with diabetes, our pancreas continues to make insulin and our tissues respond to its effects.

But each and every one of us will have four different endocrine hormones that decline steadily and predictably with age. These are human growth hormone, DHEA, melatonin, and the major sex hormones, testosterone in men and estrogen in women. The rate at which these hormones decline differs from person to person. By and large, the drop is drastic. A normal adult will have lost more than 80 percent of at least three of these hormones by the time he/she reaches his or her late seventies.

Studies have shown that these declining hormones are at particularly low levels among the inhabitants of nursing homes and in victims of heart attacks, strokes, senility, and cancer. Even before we consider the question of whether hormone replacement for all these missing natural chemicals can extend life, it seems obvious that the millions of individuals who make it into their eighties and nineties would be living far more comfortable and competent lives if their hormone levels were closer to what they had been when they were young adults. We consider quality of life to be just as important as longevity.

Some scientists have speculated that the loss of these hormones may be a necessary adaptation to the increasing weakness and inefficiency of our aging metabolism. Perhaps as our bodies get older it would become too physically stressful to deal with hormone levels that were meant for young people. We'll explore that possibility in depth when we come to discuss supplementation with estrogen, testosterone, DHEA, and human growth hormone. All that needs to be said for the moment is that clinical experience and many scientific research studies on replacing those hormones in the elderly indicate that any potential risk involved in hormone supplementation is small when measured against the well-established advantages. And those advantages are of such a nature that they both improve the quality of life and also increase the probability of living longer.

For instance, among the most common and tragic causes of disability and death in the elderly are bone fractures, particularly broken hips. Yet we now know that estrogen supplementation dramatically decreases bone loss in women, the sex that is most at risk. Growth hormone also appears to increase bone density in both sexes, while the increased muscle strength and alertness that it produces, together with improved balance and coordination, are also important in preventing falls, the most common cause of bone fractures in the elderly.

DHEA and melatonin may be equally significant for maintaining quality of life in an older body. Moreover, there is now a flood of evidence showing that—in addition to all their other benefits—these hormones deliver formidable reinforcements to the immune system. As you grow older, your immune system is, frankly, slowly dying. This can be reversed. As little as five years ago, no one suspected such a reversal was possible.

I wrote this survey of our endocrine glands to give you a sense of the big picture. Now it's time to look at the pro-longevity hormones one by one.

CHAPTER THREE

Human Growth Hormone: The Body's Maintenance and Repair Hormone

SO WE ARE GOING TO GROW OLD. THAT IS CERTAIN. IS IT ALSO certain that we will grow old in exactly the same way that human beings have since prehistoric times? As the Romans did, and the Greeks? As medieval kings did, and as millionaires have done in spite of their millions? You know what I mean. Frail. Our steps more hesitant. And in our hearts a well-founded fear that any little elevation in the pavement or dip in the road will send us sprawling. Tired, oh, so tired.

In spite of efforts to propagandize for the golden years, old age has really not been that pretty. Not in the past, and not even today with all of our comforts. It has been said that youth is wasted on the young; well, experience and money are often wasted on the old because they don't have the energy to do anything with them.

What we now know is that much of what is called old age is a deficiency state, much like a vitamin deficiency. As we age, we develop age-related hormonal deficiencies. As a physician, it startles and saddens me to consider all the thousands of elderly patients who have come to me over the years suffering from the utter depletion of old age. I was able to help many of them, no doubt about it. But if I had known then what I know now, I could have done much more. Nowadays, because of the pro-longevity hormones, I can often turn their lives completely around.

Unfortunately there are probably no more than a few hundred physicians in the United States at present who are routinely using a full spectrum of hormonal replacement therapy—not just the commonly prescribed female hormones—to rejuvenate the old.

Can there be some danger in taking hormones? Should caution be exercised in prescribing them? Yes, certainly. As you'll see, most of the hormones discussed in this book do have at least some potential for causing harm to at least some of the people who would otherwise be reasonable candidates for taking them. It wouldn't be the smartest of moves to take human growth hormone, DHEA, testosterone, or estrogen without the guidance of a physician—which is why they're prescription items. At the same time, when a prudent approach guided by lab tests is used, it strikes me that no great abundance of common sense is necessary to see that the danger for the average eighty-year-old of sinking toward senility and death—or, at least, the nursing home—is far more immediate and acute than the risk of side effects from the judicious replacement of deficient hormones.

When Americans realize that much of what we now call old age is reversible, will they stand by and allow it to remain unreversed? I wouldn't bet on it. They will want to maintain their quality of life for as long as possible. As a private citizen, I certainly don't intend to allow old age to creep up on me any faster than absolutely necessary. As a doctor who has been watching the hormone revolution take its baby steps during the past decade, I know that old age is no longer invincible. We have shot gaping holes in it. We can not only reverse the process of aging but to some extent we can actually delay the onset of aging. I don't know whether Mother Nature approves, but even she is going to have to adapt.

The next three chapters will discuss the most startling, really awe-inspiring of all the replacement hormones: Human Growth Hormone (HGH). It is also the most expensive, the most difficult to obtain, and one of the most controversial. But very ordinary, healthy people are beginning to take it purely to fight off old age. Let's look at one of them.

Tim Wallace

Tim Wallace, a seventy-three-year-old businessman, is the managing partner supervising the building of two hundred houses on a hundred rolling acres in Virginia. When that enterprise began a year and a half ago, Tim wondered if he had bitten off more than he could chew. His energy level had been slowly sagging for about a decade. This would be his last big project. Would he have the strength for it?

> I was full of enthusiasm, but pretty soon I had to admit I wasn't the man I used to be. I'd work hard in the morning, but by afternoon I'd be exhausted. Often I'd have to lie down on the office couch for an hour or two and tell my secretary to hold my calls. I began to organize the job around my fatigue. And it only got worse. After a couple of months, I decided I was the most exhausted man alive.

I saw Tim in my office in June 1995 and suggested that he might want to try human growth hormone (or HGH, as we'll often abbreviate it.) He had already begun taking DHEA, which had produced some improvement—but not enough. Now, I measured his blood levels of somatomedin-C (also called Insulin-like Growth Factor-1), a byproduct of growth hormone and the best laboratory test to use as an indicator of growth hormone (HGH) levels. Tim's level, although extremely low by the standards of a young adult, was not surprising in a man his age. Soon after the tests were done, Tim began taking injections* of HGH four times a week. Two months passed, and he noticed he had more energy. After he'd been on growth hormone replacement therapy for four months he simply wasn't fatigued anymore. "It's pretty amazing," Tim remarked some time later. "I have more muscle strength, in my legs especially, and my body fat is shrinking. Now that I've been on growth hormone for eight months, I find that when I squeeze the fat around my abdomen, I can't get a handful. I need less sleep. But the greatest change is simply what I suppose you'd call general vitality—I'm much stronger, much more alive, I've got more energy now than I've had since my forties. People who meet me for the first time can't believe it when I tell them my age.

"You know, I don't think I'm going to retire after all."

I marvel at Tim's appearance, his energy, his youthful delight in what's happening to him, and I marvel as well because I know I'm seeing a phenomenon new to the human race: the years rolling backward. Tim has bought himself extra years of vital life.

A SORT OF MIRACLE

Let's look again at the study conducted by Dr. Daniel Rudman at the Medical College of Wisconsin, which I mentioned in the first chapter.[1] Dr. Rudman had been investi-

---

*HGH is the only hormone discussed in this book that *must* be injected—a minor inconvenience in light of its benefits. Usually a fold of fat is pulled up on the abdomen or thigh and the needle is slipped in. The needle is quite tiny (27 gauge), and the injection is not particularly painful.

gating human growth hormone for some years and was already prominent in the field. He was about to become a bit of a legend.

Rudman was aware of a number of medical studies showing that children, rodents, and human adults who suffer from a deficiency in growth hormone secretion tended to experience loss of lean body mass (muscle) and expansion of adipose tissue (fat). They were weaker and fatter than they ought to be. But when given replacement doses of growth hormone, these alterations in body composition were readily reversed—in children, in rats, and in full-grown, older men and women.

Surely, Dr. Rudman reasoned, it could not be coincidence that these are also the effects naturally produced by aging and in more or less direct proportion to the decline of growth hormone that is simultaneously occurring. Decreased muscle mass, increased fat deposition, thinner skin, and—invisible but crucial—shrinkage and decreasing functionality of major internal organs all occur in the second half of life. In most people they only occur to a significant extent after the age of forty, which is just when HGH production begins to taper off more sharply. An average woman's body is 35 percent fat at age thirty and 53 percent by the time she's eighty. Similar changes occur in men, and, in both sexes, there's a corresponding decline in muscle. It would be quite surprising if there were not a causal connection between these changes and the decline of growth hormone, since one thing that studies have definitely shown is that growth hormone causes the breakdown of fat and promotes the synthesis of protein, our bodies' major building block.

The building up of healthy tissue, especially lean muscle mass, is called anabolism, and its destruction and eventual disintergration is called catabolism. (The combination of anabolism and catabolism, along with all the other chemical processes in the body, is called metabolism.) It is a medical truism to say that the first half of life is anabolic and the second half catabolic. What if a leading cause of this process was an abundance of HGH from childhood until early adulthood and a progressive deficiency from then on?

Rudman and his associates decided to take twenty-one healthy men from sixty-one to eighty-one years of age with somatomedin-C concentrations in the lower 30 percent of what's normal and divide them into two groups. Twelve men received three injections of growth hormone per week for six months, and nine men received no treatment. All the men remained healthy. Nonetheless, the differences between the treated and untreated groups after six months was startling. The twelve men on HGH increased the amount of muscle on their bodies by 8.8 percent and decreased their total amount of fat by 14.4 percent. Their skin thickness increased 7.1 percent and their vertebral bone density 1.6 percent. The untreated men showed no significant changes.

What had happened to these twelve men on growth hormone was also visible to the naked eye. Physically, as best anyone could tell, these men had become younger. I know that's a crude, seat-of-the-pants method of estimating age. But isn't it what we all do when we first meet someone?

Standing in a bathing suit on the edge of the sea, many of the subjects of Rudman's experiement now looked five to ten years younger than they had six months before—at any rate, from the neck down. Much of their flab was gone, their muscles were better defined, they were altogether harder, leaner specimens. Achieving this had required no exercise at all, which is a clear contradiction of the normal route to good conditioning. They had simply changed. Age had run effortlessly backward for them, just as, in the normal process of life, age runs effortlessly forward.

Rudman published his results in July 1990 in the *New England Journal of Medicine*, and like a time bomb, the possibility of a genuine reversal of the aging process began to form in the minds of hundreds of scientists around the globe. What was going on here?

JUST WHAT IS GROWTH HORMONE?

Created in the anterior (frontal) portion of the pituitary gland, growth hormone is a small proteinlike hormone (peptide) with a known sequence of 191 amino acids. It is chemically rather similar to insulin. Secreted in very brief pulses during the early hours of sleep, growth hormone remains in the circulatory system for only a few minutes and is therefore difficult to measure. The body takes much of it up into the liver and converts some of it into somatomedin-C, another small peptide hormone formerly referred to as Insulin-Like Growth Factor-1—"IGF-1," for short. Somatomedin-C is responsible for some of the activity of growth hormone in the body. Moreover, since somatomedin-C exists in the circulatory system for twenty-four to thirty-six hours and is therefore more stable than growth hormone, a laboratory test for its levels in the blood gives a more reliable indication of total growth hormone production by the pituitary gland.

A normal level of somatomedin-C in a young adult is approximately 300 to 450 nanograms per milliliter, abbreviated ng/ml—some laboratories use different units of measurement. Men and women older than fifty usually have levels ranging from 200 down to as low as 30 or less. Depending on body size and also on how low the initial level was, four units of growth hormone injected weekly, usually in four injections—one unit each time—taken on different days, will sometimes (theoretically) bring those levels up to between 250 and 350. In older adults, even when levels stabilize at 150 to 200, patients report noticeable enhancement of physical endurance and alleviation of many of the "symptoms" of aging.

Having said that, I must confess that, in practice, the interpretation of somatomedin-C measurements has had severe limitations. I always take a baseline measurement to find out if pretreatment levels are high or low. I advise the rare older patient whose levels are still high that HGH may not be worth the effort and expense. With the person whose levels are very low, I have come to expect more rapid clinical improvement. However, I have found that follow-up measurements of somatomedin-C often do not correlate well with the clinical benefit received. Frequently, patients who report great improvements on HGH do not show much increase in somatomedin-C levels. And not uncommonly, patients whose somatomedin-C levels increase substantially do not seem to experience correspondingly dramatic benefits. Consequently, I no longer fully rely on routine follow-up testing of somatomedin-C after therapy has begun. Its effectiveness as a guide to therapy is not nearly as great as a close and accurate observation of actual physical and symptomatic improvements in the individual man or woman being treated. In other words, I treat the patient, not the laboratory report.

Effects of Growth Hormone

During adolescence, when growth is most rapid, production of growth hormone is also very high. However, once growth is complete, HGH must still be present throughout life at the lower maintenance levels, represented by the numbers above, to maintain physical and mental health and well-being. Tissue repair; cell replacement; healing; organ integrity; bone strength; brain function; enzyme production; and integrity of hair, nails, and skin all require the ongoing availability of adequate growth hormone. Without such a supply, these anabolic processes are crippled.

In childhood, growth hormone controls a major miracle—growth itself. Children with a pituitary deficiency of growth hormone are therefore incapable of normal growth. And until HGH became available—first in small amounts in the 1970s and then in unlimited quantities after 1985—such children inevitably reached adulthood as dwarfs.

Once we reach adulthood and our growth stops, the secretion of growth hormone begins to fall. For some decades, however, it remains at a level sufficient to maintain a healthy adult body. It cannot be emphasized too forcefully that the term "growth hormone" is misleading. Growth is only one of the hormone's functions; "growth" hormone is an all-purpose maintenance and repair hormone. It is absolutely essential for a high quality of life.

Unfortunately, its production declines inexorably as we age. Eventually we are flat-out *deficient*. No other word is appropriate. Averaged out over a lifetime, the declines will be about 10 to 15 percent per decade. By the age of sixty it is not uncommon to measure growth hormone decline of 75 percent or more from the abundant levels normally seen in twenty-five-year-olds. By causing a significant reversal of the weakness and fraility of age, Rudman's experiment— which has been repeated since by other investigators— seems to confirm logical expectations. Without HGH we cannot enjoy the physical strength of our earlier years; with it we are suddenly and startlingly reinvested with physical power and a sizable proportion of our youth-like vigor.

Won't Run on Empty

If the decline of growth hormone is so debilitating, what happens when there's none at all? The most common cause of such a dead stop is a pituitary tumor necessitating surgery.

In 1989, Douglas Harvill was a vigorous and relatively youthful sixty-three-year-old Virginia businessman. He had no apparent health problems until one day he was diagnosed with a malignant tumor on his pituitary gland. The cancer was excised, along with the pituitary gland itself. The operation was a success, and, following a short convalescence, Harvill resumed his life. He was given hormonal replacements for all the hormones for which the pituitary is responsible, with the exception of growth hormone. That is the normal protocol in a case like his. Growth hormone (largely through the efforts of the Food and Drug Administration) has been carefully restricted in its use to growth hormone deficient children. Doctors who wish to purchase HGH in the United States have been forced to submit written case records to the manufacturer, naming the child to whom they intend to administer the hormone, and including growth charts and blood-test results to confirm dwarfism caused by growth hormone deficiency.

For Douglas Harvill, the result of this restriction by the FDA was that he suddenly discovered what a colossal obstacle fatigue can be.

> I had no strength at all. For the first time that I could ever remember, I hated to get up in the morning. I was sleeping an average of twelve hours a night and then two or three hours after I woke I'd get so exhausted that I had to go back to bed again. I was absolutely worthless. I'd always been physically very active, but now I found that no matter how much I forced myself to exercise I could build no muscle. Month by month and year by year I was growing weaker.

Douglas began reading up on growth hormone and discovered that there were European studies showing that average human survival after the removal of the pituitary gland was only ten years. In older people it could be considerably less with cardiovascular problems high amongst the causes of mortality. He was determined to obtain growth hormone, but the obstacles in his path were considerable. Supplementation with HGH for adults, even adults who were chronically deficient—or, in his case, totally deprived—was not yet standard medical practice (and to a large extent still isn't). It took Douglas Harvill over two years, with my help and the support of his endocrinologist, to get his supply of growth hormone.

The results for him were more dramatic than they would be for an ordinary person.

> Within ten days after my first injection, my strength and endurance had increased 50 percent. I could literally see myself recovering day by day. I went to my endocrinologist and said, "You're going to think I'm making this up." But he believed me. It only took a few months to gain back almost everything I had lost over two years. My coordination and balance dramatically improved. My muscles started coming back. All my energy came back. The difference was phenomenal.

This enormous improvement was achieved by administering just one unit of growth hormone four days per week.

Douglas Harvill is now sixty-nine years old and enjoying a retirement that I suppose is not for everyone. Certainly it's different from our normal image of old age. Douglas had always wanted to ride a motorcycle. He now owns three Harley-Davidsons and, in the cool of the morning, can more often than not be found roaring along the twisty Shenandoah Valley roads.

It's What Makes You Strong!

One of the striking things about HGH is its ability to produce improvements in people who certainly haven't reached old age yet.

Consider Chad Strether, a Minnesota engineer who at fifty-six is still in the midst of an outstandingly vigorous and energetic life. Chad runs three or four times weekly and gets plenty of other forms of physical exercise. He's something of a computer buff, a lover of classical music, and a man whose wife still considers him a hunk. (So they both say.)

He should have no complaints, right? Well, he had a little one. Age was creeping up, and he was tracking it because, being an engineer, he was a man dedicated to precision, with a habit of keeping careful numerical records. He had noticed two things about his running: it wasn't nearly as much fun as it used to be, and he certainly wasn't doing it as well. His times on his two and three mile runs were going steadily down. He'd also noticed that now, when he ran two consecutive days, he did more poorly the second day. It used to be that he did better. And, though he watched his diet, slowly but surely, fifteen pounds of middle-aged spread had attached itself to his middle.

Chad also felt that mentally he wasn't quite as sharp as he used to be. Creative solutions didn't come as easily for engineering problems. He wasn't as quick at games. And he didn't like any of this. In January 1996, he found a doctor who prescribed him HGH. By the end of February, our meticulous, record-keeping engineer was observing changes.

He was clocking himself running—at times that he hadn't seen in years. He sensed that his balance and coordination had improved, and his running regimen was no longer torture for his muscles. His home exercise routine involves situps, pushups, and a series of rows on a rowing machine. Chad times it with a stopwatch. His best time in the previous year had been 7 minutes 26 seconds. After five weeks of HGH, he hit 7:05, then 6:54, 6:42. His weight fell eight pounds by April.

Chad also noticed that he played computer games more efficiently. (Yes, he times that, too.) At the same time, his intuitive impression—hard to measure exactly—was that he was becoming more creative in his work.

Chad was also excited by one other unexpected change. Classical music has always been a big part of his life. Now when he goes to concerts, which he does three or four times a month, he notices that, "I'm hearing high notes that I haven't heard in years."

I'm impressed by these changes. If they don't seem as extensive as the changes we've pointed out in older individuals that's because Chad was actually in tip-top physical and mental state.

Let's look at one other example, this time in an even younger, but very different man.

Ben Herzen, a New Jersey restaurateur and nightclub owner, started taking growth hormone at the age of fifty-three simply because he noticed he wasn't functioning any longer at the extraordinarily high level he was accustomed to. Ben owns nine nightclubs, is a city council member, a prominent figure in countless political organizations and charities, and a man who has worked hard and played hard since before he was old enough to vote. "How do you do it?" friends would ask him about his very active life. Ben would smile and shrug.

Now, however, he was beginning to notice the natural signs of middle age—the desire to sit at home with his feet up in front of the television set was suddenly becoming greater than the urge to go out to dinner or make it to that city council meeting. His hyperactive business life wasn't as easy to handle as it used to be. One night on television he saw a program that talked about human growth hormone and people who were going down to Mexico to get it. Intrigued, Ben spoke to his doctor, had his blood levels of somatomedin-C checked, and eventually obtained a supply of HGH for his personal use in this country.

He started taking it in March of 1995, and by June noticed that he was starting to feel a little different. By September, he had no doubt at all that something had happened. Such a gradual, progressive improvement during the first six to twelve months of HGH therapy is not unusual.

> Everything was just working better. It was as if some-thing inside me was different. When I took a vacation in Mexico last year all I wanted to do was sit on the beach and read a book. This year I went out and swam for two hours. I had gotten fifteen years of energy back. My legs and arms work better; I feel more coordinated; my mus-cles are hard again, and when I spent an afternoon at a friend's swimming pool, he asked me if I had joined a health club. I told him what I'd really done. I don't think growth hormone is a miracle drug. It's just replacing what I'd lost. But that's enough. I think everybody over fifty should be on growth hormone.

Should everyone over fifty be on growth hormone? In the present state of our knowledge, I would never suggest that, and, as you'll see in the next chapter, there are some people who do experience side effects. HGH is too potent to be taken incautiously, indiscriminately, or without a physi-cian's guidance as if it were some sort of an injectable aspirin. But I believe it's already clear that, taken under the supervision of a physician, HGH is going to be the most remarkable answer to aging that the human race has devised so far.

Are millions of people going to be taking it soon? The answer to that may have been given by Edward Chein, M.D., of the Life Extension Foundation, when he said to me that this was a "national security issue." By which he meant that the U.S. government couldn't afford to let it be known that growth hormone works for anything other than growth-deficient children. Twenty million elderly people taking growth hormone at a cost of more than $10,000 per person per annum represents $200 billion yearly added to the nation's Medicare bill. That's the amount of money that Congress and the President spent much of 1995 and 1996 talking with great anguish and tumult about cutting from the federal budget over *seven* years. If the Food and Drug Administration is violently opposed to growth hormone use in adults, they have sound political reasons. It seems that our national health-care policy has degenerated to the rationing of limited resources. At the moment, this country cannot afford the fountain of youth. Translation: people who want it are going to have to pay for it themselves.

THE WHOLE LINEUP

Okay, growth hormone is impressive, no doubt about it. Here are some of the things that carefully conducted medical studies—most of them conducted in the six years since Dr. Daniel Rudman opened Pandora's box—have shown it can do:

- Increases muscle
- Decreases fat
- Increases skin thickness
- Smooths out skin wrinkles in some people
- Improves exercise tolerance
- Improves pulmonary function in people with chronic lung disorders
- Increases restorative REM sleep
- Increases energy and endurance
- Protects mental function and appears to help in the treatment of neurological and mental disorders such as Alzheimer's and Parkinson's diseases, and multiple sclerosis
- Enhances mental alertness and memory
- Increases the size of the thymus, the body's principal immune system gland
- Increases natural killer cell lymphocyte activity, a measure of immune system function
- Greatly increases longevity in animal studies

- Causes weight gain in frail elderly
- Causes some regrowth and regeneration of organs (liver, kidneys, and spleen) that have shrunk with age
- Normalizes serum cholesterol levels
- Causes hair and nails to improve in strength and appearance
- Speeds healing after surgery and trauma
- Greatly improves the quality of life in AIDS patients

These are the effects of this natural hormone *given to people at doses calculated to maintain the body's supply at the levels normally present during young adulthood*. The quantities used are extraordinarily minute. A year's supply of growth hormone in concentrated form would be smaller than an average vitamin C tablet.

Growth hormone may not be as explosive as enriched uranium, but its potency within the human body is, I dare say, fully appropriate to the nuclear age.

CHAPTER FOUR

The Body of Evidence

YOU KNOW NOW WHAT MOST SCIENTISTS AND ACADEMIC endocrinologists at medical centers around the world are aware of: growth hormone significantly—in many elderly people, vastly—increases muscular strength and energy. And the image of a frail oldster suddenly transformed into Arnold Schwarzenegger (well, not quite!) is, I suppose, sufficiently startling to make this hormone's name and fame.

However, this book is about longevity. If all HGH did was add on extra muscle, its stature as a pro-longevity hormone would be limited. Such a physical improvement can certainly minister to an older person's comfort and sense of competence, but I'd be surprised if, on average, it gave him more than an extra year or two of life. There are so many other ways besides muscle loss in which we age. Some are extremely significant to our health and quality of life. How much of what we call heart disease is aging? To what extent is bone loss a direct response to depleted hormones? Why does mental function decline in a significant proportion of the elderly? Why does an infection that would only cause an eighteen-year-old a feverish, uncomfortable evening kill an eighty-year-old? Let's go through that list in reverse order. HGH appears to be a major player in every single one of these conditions.

THE WANING OF THE IMMUNE SYSTEM

If they could afford it and didn't mind the isolation, very old people would have reason to live inside sterile bubbles like those rare, sad children who are born without immune systems. Somewhere between the ages of seventy and eighty-five, the human immune system takes a nosedive, and far too many of us go down with it. Enter HGH again.

Growth hormone's changes aren't only the ones found rippling just beneath the surface of the suddenly tighter and tauter skin. There's something more profound than that. *We now have every reason to think HGH supplementation will radically upgrade the quality of the aging immune system!*

Now it's possible you don't find the immune system very exciting. You may take it for granted—just an old, dull part of your body that does its job when you catch that winter cold. However, the truth is that it's the premier instrument of your survival. You wouldn't last long without a skin to cover the outside of you, and you wouldn't live a whole lot longer without an immune system to protect the inside of you. The world is a dangerous place filled with bacterial lions and tigers and viral dragons out to get you. There are sharklike parasites that long to munch on your juicy interior and hungry yeasts that would like nothing better than to grow at your expense. So to live is to live in peril. These dangerous microbial wanderers assault you daily. Yet so fantastically powerful is your immune system, that most days you feel quite healthy and aren't even aware of the battles being fought on your behalf by your lymphocytes and phagocytes and killer cells. In Chapter Seven, I'll explain in greater detail the highly discplined and warlike system that guards our physical integrity.

For now, it's sufficient that you accept its supreme importance and realize that it's a scientific fact that immune response declines with advancing age. And once we've reached our seventh or eighth decades, the decline is likely to be quite profound. This immunological falling-off is a major contributing cause of the increase in cancers, in autoimmune disorders such as rheumatoid arthritis, and, of course, in simple viral and bacterial infections—everything from the common cold to full-blown pneumonia. In extreme old age, the immune system has a difficult time dealing with even the simplest biological hazards of life. At some point in time, people who are fortunate enough to live that long arrive at an immunological crisis point: they're simply waiting for the first haphazard puff of infection or growth of malignancy to lay them low. How does one go from the incredibly hearty immune system of the adolescent to the frail and crumbling defense network of the senior citizen?

In many scientist's opinion, the first, and eventually most significant negative change begins as early as puberty. Our thymus gland, the source of the T-cell lymphocytes (a form of white blood cell) that lead the immune-system charge when infection and unwanted intrusions of any kind take place, begins to shrink. Important thymic cells are replaced by fat tissue, leading to decreased thymic hormone secretion. By old age, the thymus has nearly disappeared—and so has our immune system. Naturally immunologists have wondered whether this shrinkage of the thymus is controlled by a biological clock or is the result of age-associated imbalances in the endocrine system.

It has been noticed that thymic shrinkage and growth hormone decline begin more or less simultaneously in adolescence. Of course, this could be coincidental. But research in the 1960s showed that the injection of middle-aged animals with pituitary extracts could augment thymic size. That was definitely suggestive.

In the last ten years, we've gone beyond coincidence or mere suggestion. It has been demonstrated experimentally that mice, rats, and dogs, all of whom suffer thymic shrinkage with age and consequent immune decline in a manner very similar to humans, are all capable of regenerating their thymus glands. HGH is the key hormone that does it.

Dr. Keith Kelley, a researcher at the Indiana University School of Medicine, made one of the first experimental demonstrations in 1986. He took sixteen- to twenty-two-month-old female rats—this is the beginning of old age in rats—and implanted young pituitary cells under their skin. A control group of similarly aged rats was untreated. After two months of treatment both groups of rats were killed. Only remnants of the thymus gland were found in the control rats. The treated rats had larger, functional thymus glands and the numbers of T-cells produced by their splenocytes (a type of white blood cell) were two to five times that found in the untreated rats. Kelley concluded that it was possible to regenerate normal thymic tissue and reverse the natural loss of immunity.[1]

In 1987 Dr. William Monroe did a similar study with dogs and, after giving them growth-hormone therapy, found that "the thymuses of growth-hormone-treated dogs regenerated, resembling thymic tissue of young dogs."[2]

These were fairly short-term studies and though they showed that a thymus gland shrunken by age has an astonishing capacity to recover, they didn't yet show what effect such treatment would have on longevity. In 1991 David Khansari and Thomas Gustad of North Dakota State University completed a lengthier study on mice. The results were truly startling. Taking fifty-two mice who had reached the age (seventeen months) at which healthy, well-cared for mice will begin to die off, they divided them into two groups of twenty-six mice each, one group receiving growth hormone for thirteen weeks.

In that time span, sixteen control mice (61 percent) died, whereas only two of the hormone-treated mice (7 percent) expired. After a break of four weeks, HGH therapy was continued for another six weeks. One more of the HGH mice died. But, by the end of this period, the mice in the control group no longer existed. Dead to the last mouse! The surviving growth-hormone-treated mice had already passed beyond the outer limits of mouse longevity. And it was found that their immune production of T-cells was comparable to that of young mice. Not wishing to overstate their results, the two researchers modestly concluded that the mortality curve obtained "suggests that long-term low-dose growth hormone treatment prolongs life expectancy."[3]

The truth is that the only other substance that has had a similar effect in the extension of longevity is melatonin, which coincidentally has also shown a capacity to regenerate the thymus gland.

IN HUMANS?

We already have evidence that growth hormone will indeed stimulate one kind of immunity in people. A study was conducted at the University of New Mexico School of Medicine on older women with low levels of human growth hormone.[4] The researchers were intrigued by the correlation of two facts. First, that in both animals and humans a deficiency in growth hormone is associated with an impairment in natural killer (NK) cell activity. Second, that a decrease in NK activity occurs naturally with aging.

NK cells have somewhat different targets from the T-cells that are produced by the thymus. The T-cells are preprogrammed to respond to specific antigens, and the victims of their assault are most often invading viruses and bacteria. Natural killer cells choose cancer cells as their primary targets, especially blood-borne metastatic cancer cells in the process of spreading.

Until scientists worked out the function of NK cells, they had often assumed that the body has little natural defense against cancer. If we didn't all die of it relatively quickly, that had to be because malignancies were rather rare malfunctions of the body. Nowadays, we realize that cancer cells are anything but rare. The billions of cells in the human body with their trillions of daily interactions inevitably produce rogue cells all the time. If we can go for many decades—and the majority of us for a lifetime—without contracting cancer, that's because our bodies are programmed to promptly and decisively destroy these renegades.

Recent research indicates that NK cells are designed to sense any cell that is dividing at an abnormally rapid rate—which is the exact characteristic of a cancer. NK cells go directly to such a site of abnormality; attach themselves to the suspect cell; and, acting as judge, jury, and executioner all in one, give it such a walloping dose of chemical toxicity that the offending malignant cell promptly croaks. Immunologists now believe that without these superb and necessary assassins, we would very quickly become statistics on the national cancer charts. Which is exactly what happens to a large percentage of AIDS patients as their natural killer cell counts go down.

The researchers in New Mexico were aware that growth hormone declines naturally with age as does NK activity. Taking twelve older women in otherwise good health but with low HGH levels, they gave growth hormone to six for fourteen days while leaving the other six untreated. At the end of the experiment, the growth-hormone-treated women had increased their level of natural-killer-cell activity by 20 percent.

Growth Hormone Against
Skin Cancer

With great interest I've observed in my patients a phenomenon new to science. Patients with early skin cancer lesions on the face and hands have occasionally found these minor malignancies vanishing without surgery after a period on HGH. A friend and colleague of mine, James P. Frackelton, M.D., of Cleveland, Ohio, has had similar experiences with his growth hormone patients. In one case a man with a squamous cell carcinoma, one of the faster spreading varieties of skin cancer, was completely cured without surgical or other treatment.

Dr. Frackelton is fortunate enough to have an excellent clinical laboratory next to his office. Measuring immune function before and after growth hormone replacement therapy, he has found consistent increases in natural killer cell lymphocyte (NK) counts in his elderly patients, in some cases by as much as 300 percent.

An interesting side issue that this study raises is the relationship between HGH, obesity, immune system function, and cancer. It is well known that obese women tend to have lower HGH levels, impaired natural killer cell activity, and a higher risk of cancer. Is it their weight that increases their cancer risk or is it actually depressed immune function resulting from lower levels of HGH?

And what about the thymus regeneration I paid so much attention to in animals? There is evidence here, too, though not so much as we're likely to have in a few years when a number of current studies I'll tell you about in the next chapter bear fruit. Dr. Edmund Chein of the Life Extension Foundation has reported some degree of thymic regeneration within four weeks of beginning HGH supplementation in humans. An interesting early (1987) study conducted by scientists at the University of Bologna in Italy also found that giving large doses of intravenous arginine, an amino acid that is known to provoke the secretion of growth hormone, produced almost a full recovery in the secretion of thymic hormones even at a very old age.[5]

As this research continues to pile up, it is going to become harder and harder to avoid the conclusion that one of the chief antagonists of the elderly—depressed immune function—is treatable.

Now let's think about thinking.

Bolstering the Brain?

There's little doubt that one of the most feared results of aging is a decline in our mental function. What would it profit us to live longer, if our headpieces were no longer in functional shape, our thoughts grown incoherent, our speech fumbling and slow, our old memories fading, and our capacity to form new memories nearly nonexistent? And I do not even speak of the horrors of that most severe form of senile dementia, the rightly dreaded Alzheimer's disease. And since by some estimates at least a third of eighty-five-year-olds display signs of Alzheimer's, any book on longevity that fails to consider ways and means of protecting mental function is surely sadly lacking.

Not all of the evidence is in by any means, but many scientists now believe growth hormone is a powerful tool in the preservation of brain function, memory, and intellect. Let's consider for a moment the way brain cells function. It's quite different from the way things work in the rest of your body.

Approximately every three years 90 percent of the 100 trillion cells in the human body are made anew in a constant process of cell death and replacement. Only in the brain and nervous system are the original cells retained forever. These nerve cells are called neurons, and the average human brain contains many trillions of them. That's your working intellectual capital. You won't get more of it. There are no undifferentiated precursor cells waiting to develop into mature nerve cells. For the rest of your life, you'll dance with what you brought to the ball.

Our neurons form a web of billions of trillions of interconnections—called synapses—so vast that our brain puts to shame the most sophisticated manmade computer ever built. Neurons grow long filamentous extensions like telephone wires that connect to myriad other neurons in the brain. The final leap from neuron to neuron is made by tiny molecules (neurotransmitters) specially fitted for their task. Our brain's neurons also extend via connections similar to telephone switchboards to every organ and tissue throughout the body.

Whenever we have a new experience or learn a new fact, new connections are woven. This process is supported by small protein molecules called nerve growth factor (NGF). A steady supply of nerve growth factor is necessary to maintain the connections that have been built up in our brains. Once a sufficient number of these connections are lost—or once an excessively high percentage of our irreplaceable neurons die due to illness, free radical oxidation, drugs, alcohol, environmental poisoning, stroke, or blows to the head—the result is mental inefficiency, possibly a very measurable decline in your mental functioning, perhaps eventually senility or Alzheimer's. The exact processes that are taking place within our brain to cause this damage are somewhat mysterious. But, since we know it occurs, it would be quite sufficient, for the moment, to learn how to protect ourselves from it.

An important discovery of recent years is that growth hormone and its byproduct somatomedin-C can also act as nerve growth factors. If they too support the functioning of the central nervous system, then growth hormone's decline may be in part responsible for the mental decline that many people experience with age. Certainly, as you're about to see, replacement of HGH can have startling effects on people with many forms of neurological disorder—not just mental but physical as well.

Repair of Nervous System Injury

A doctor in Montana telephoned me recently to describe a patient of his, a man in his fifties afflicted with a progressive form of paralysis that ran in his family. By the time growth hormone therapy was started, he was no longer able to walk and confined to a wheelchair. Within a few months he was again walking unassisted. In the year that has passed since then, he has continued to hold off the decline that his heriditary genetic defect seems to have planned for him.

This was extremely interesting to me because it corresponded to effects I was seeing when growth hormone was applied to other neurological disorders.

David Webster, a friend of my daughter, had had a car accident in August 1994. Initially he seemed to have suffered only severe soft tissue damage, but soon he began to display further symptoms. His eyes totally lost their peripheral vision and had hardly any depth of field. He had severe pains in his back. He was tremendously fatigued and began to suffer balance problems. Going to some of the top neurologists in southern California, he was given a series of MRIs, and—three months after his accident— David Webster was diagnosed with multiple sclerosis. Six very characteristic MRI lesions seen on his brain made the diagnosis definite. Though seldom reported, this is a medical pattern that neurologists are quite familar with: MS is frequently triggered in the aftermath of some form of severe physical trauma.

The exact cause of MS is still not known, but it is widely agreed that the immune system is involved in an attack on the myelin sheaths that surround each nerve fiber. Those sheaths act just like the insulation on an electrical wire. When the sheath is destroyed by a disordered immunity, the nerve fibers short circuit and cease to conduct messages to and from the neurons. It therefore makes good sense to think that a substance that improves the functioning of the immune system might also improve the symptoms of multiple sclerosis.

David, who at the age of forty-two is a successful international trader, had an extraordinarily demanding work schedule, which his doctors were advising him to curtail. He was in severe pain and was barely ambulatory, his hands constantly shook, and he was now spending most of his time in bed, conducting his business from a supine position. He had been put on a full cocktail of modern medications—muscle relaxants, pain killers, and sleeping medications. He was diagnosed as having one of the most severe, rapidly progressive forms of MS, and his prospects were not good. Nonetheless, David was not giving up, and he contiued to travel whenever his business made it necessary. On a trip to China, he received several months of hands-on treatment (literally, for this was Oriental medicine) from a physician used by officials high in the Chinese government, and he showed some definite improvement.

Back in the United States, however, he continued to regress. I had advised him to eat a diet high in fresh vegetables and excluding all sugar, dairy products, red meat, and wheat. He also began taking DHEA. Real improvement began, however, when one of his neurologists, at my suggestion, agreed to put David on growth hormone. He was eventually taking much larger doses than would be used for purely anti-aging purposes, at a cost of two thousand dollars a month. His blood levels of somatomedin-C tripled. And his improvement was startling. His eyesight and coordination greatly improved. He had far less fatigue and greater endurance for physical activity. He could walk reasonably well for short distances and was no longer bedbound. He was still leading a very careful lifestyle, and, if he began to overdo things, he suffered a partial relapse, but, by and large, he was a far more functional person than he had been before the start of growth hormone therapy, and this improvement has now continued for more than a year.

Will results like this be found in the treatment of other neurological disorders? Edward Chein, M.D., of the Life Extension Foundation in Palm Springs, California, has said with reference to growth hormone that "We have a therapy that can repair systems. Damage to the neurologic system resulting from age or injury can be repaired." Chaovanee Aroonsakul, M.D., of the Alzheimer's and Parkinson's Disease Diagnostic and Treatment Center in Naperville, Illinois, has discussed her own successes using growth hormone. She has been able to demonstrate the regeneration of nerve cells, restored hormonal balance, and improved functional capacity in patients with Alzheimer's disease, senile dementia, Parkinson's disease, and stroke. Dr. Aroonsakul writes that "Further experience with these methods has demonstrated their usefulness for a variety of aging-related conditions including osteoporosis, osteoarthritis, sexual dysfunction, lack of stamina, and mental and physical slowing."[6]

I find particularly interesting the fact that in her study of over three hundred patients, Dr. Aroonsakul has recorded consistently lower levels of HGH in patients with Parkinson's, MS, and stroke and a "profound deficiency" of HGH in Alzheimer's patients. In her work with Alzheimer's patients, some improvement frequently occurs within weeks after first administration of growth hormone. However, maximal benefits often require several years of ongoing treatment. This is not surprising. Growth hormone is not a miracle drug. It is a natural hormone that works by stimulating the slow rebuilding and replacement of healthy, efficient cells.

Exactly what it does for brain cells is not yet fully understood. It's probable, however, that HGH's capacity to accelerate protein synthesis is crucial. It's known that when the enzymes required for protein synthesis (and therefore for healing and continued cellular regeneration) are lacking in the brain, cellular death can occur. Dr. Aroonsakul believes that growth hormone's beneficial effects include:

- A general increase in cerebral blood flow, thereby enhancing the metabolism of brain cells
- Enhanced growth and repair of protein (anabolism) leading to increased activity of brain cells and an increase in the formation of DNA and RNA
- A revitalization of neuronal dendrites and axons

As our population ages, Alzheimer's looks more and more like an epidemic, and my conversations with leading neurologists around the country have left me with no doubt that growth hormone is going to be one of the most closely researched treatments in this growing field.

Such treatments will become all the more important if, as this book predicts, human longevity shows a very marked increase in the coming decades. Odd as it may seem, there are some indications that Alzheimer's and Parkinson's are not so much "diseases" as part of the normal process of aging. Aren't the shakiness and the clumsy steps of a typical ninety-year-old basically due to the same shortage of dopamine-producing neurons that we call Parkinson's when we find it in a fifty-year-old? Yet no one speaks of Parkinson's in regard to the ninety-year-old unless the symptoms are very advanced indeed. As for Alzheimer's, more than half of the men and women in their nineties are in at least the first stages of it. Aren't

Parkinson's and Alzheimer's therefore just part of the normal process of aging? Probably no one would have called them diseases if it wasn't that they occur in a certain percentage of people who haven't yet reached advanced old age. Instead, we'd still be calling Alzheimer's senility, and Parkinson's would be merely the characteristic tremors of extreme antiquity. I exaggerate, but only slightly.

The intriguing thing about HGH and its effect upon these neurological disorders is that what it may actually be doing is slowing the aging process in people who for one reason or another are the victims of premature aging. But if it can do this for people who have been dealt an unlucky hand in the genetic card game, then presumably it can also slow aging in the rest of us and help to ensure that we won't be slow of wit and step when we're ninety but rather pushing on vigorously toward a hundred. Certainly this is speculation but not without foundation. In addition to all its other benefits, HGH replacement therapy may eventually earn recognition as a major form of preventive medicine.

The Full Spectrum of Therapy

We've talked at length about HGH's capacity to increase energy and muscle strength, its enhancement of immune function, and its effects on the central nervous system. If those three things were all it did—and if it did them as efficiently and forcefully as the evidence indicates it does—then I suppose we would have a good and valid reason for saying that this was the most important anti-aging substance ever discovered and perhaps one of the half-dozen greatest medical breakthroughs of this medically crowded century! Very likely it is all of that.

But you remember I ended the last chapter with a list of HGH's beneficial effects. Several of them are worth discussing at greater length since they will have major signif-

Growth Hormone Promotes Healing

It seems very likely that in a few more years no one will even consider undergoing major surgery without first receiving human growth hormone injections for as many weeks or months as time allows. Astonishing improvements in healing have become commonplace in the reports of people on growth hormone.

One of my own patients, a skeptical and medically conservative forty-eight-year-old dentist named Herb Halliday, started taking HGH when his brother, a doctor, told him how much success he was having mending the broken hips of older female patients with the help of the hormone. Halliday had led a vigorously athletic life since childhood, and the price he had had to pay for pursuing half a dozen sports into middle age included two broken collarbones, knee injuries, and back injuries. Now he was set for back surgery, an operation very similar to one he had had ten years before. He began taking HGH, and when the operation was performed, he was astonished to discover that he healed much more quickly and easily this time than he had when he was a decade younger.

I had another patient who had been troubled by a gimpy knee for several years. Within a few months of starting growth hormone therapy, the problem went away. This man, who's only forty-one, has a serious hip problem. A cartilage hole in the hip socket causes him more or less continuous pain, which in a few more years may be severe enough to make him a candidate for a hip replacement. We're watching closely to see if supplemental HGH will help his body repair the cartilage. If it does, this will be an unexpected breakthrough, but not entirely surprising considering the powers of the hormone.

icance for some of my readers and some significance for almost all of you.

Loss of bone is a bane of aging. Women have taken it more to heart, for not only do they have less bone to start with, they begin losing it sooner and at a faster pace than their male counterparts. For them, ten years before the average man, the consequences of ignoring bone loss can be literally shattering. A large percentage of women in nursing homes arrive courtesy of a broken hip.

For many women, estrogen (and progesterone) replacement therapy (see Chapter Nine) can be an important part of the solution. HGH may turn out to be the other part. Rudman's original study showed a 1.7 percent increase in the bone density of the lumbar vertebrae. Though this may seem slight, bone replacement, like bone loss, accumulates over time, and Rudman's subjects were men. In another recent study, forty-two postmenopausal women with low bone mass were treated with HGH for twelve weeks. In just three months, the rate of new bone formation increased by 30 to 40 percent.[7]

In California Dr. Edmund Chein has treated scores of patients with osteoporosis with human growth hormone and has measured increases in bone density averaging 2 to 3 percent a year.[8] Since the average postmenopausal woman is losing bone at a rate approaching that, this apparently modest increase is actually not so modest, and such a reversal of fortune in the bone department is a result devoutly to be wished for.

When it comes to heart disease, the gender advantage reverses itself—men are at risk approximately a decade earlier than women. It's extremely interesting that growth hormone deficiency in adults is associated with a sharply increased risk of death from cardiovascular illness. And, of course, in old age when the highest percentage of cardiovascular illness occurs, we are all, by definition, HGH deficient.

Some of the typical physical characteristics that put older men and women at risk for blocked arteries and eventual heart attacks appear to be at least partially reversible when growth hormone levels are high. One of these is obvious enough—being overweight. But studies have shown that HGH not only reduces fat, it reduces it around the waist and abdomen. One analysis showed a 27 percent decrease in skin-fold thickness in that area after months of HGH administration. For folks in their middle years and older who are trying to avoid a heart attack, this is highly significant. So-called "upper body obesity" is firmly associated with the risk of heart disease.

The gender associations are interesting. Most men when they gain weight put it on around the chest and abdomen. This cardiovascularly unfortunate distribution correlates well with their higher heart attack risk. Women—premenopausally—gain weight mostly in their buttocks and thighs. Result: no increase in heart attack risk. After menopause, however, they, too, begin to gain weight in their upper body. How much they gain has a direct statistical association with their chance of heart disease. The closer they get to the male pattern of upper body heaviness, the more at risk they are.

In addition, in some studies, HGH replacement lowers levels of "bad" LDL cholesterol. And low blood levels of HGH are also associated with low levels of "good" HDL cholesterol. To the extent that cholesterol affects the likelihood of heart attacks—and the cholesterol theory has been somewhat exaggerated—these changes can only prove protective in the person who takes supplemental HGH. People with lower levels of HGH are definitely at greater risk for cardiovascular mishaps. In fact, ultrasound imaging has shown them to have greater thickening of blood vessel walls when compared to more normal population groups.

One final fact is easily overlooked but shouldn't be. The heart is just as much a muscle as the bicep in your arm, and, in the demands that are made on it, it's the premier muscle of the human body. Three billion beats in an average lifetime. Therefore, shouldn't it suffer adverse effects when the body's main muscle-building hormone declines? Well, I think so, and a new study of growth-hormone-deficient adults before and after supplementation with HGH certainly supports that conclusion. Dr. Antonio Cittadini and his colleagues at the Federico II University Medical School in Italy measured the cardiac impairments in eleven patients, both at rest and during exercise. After light to moderate exercise, the patients complained of weakness. Their systolic blood pressure (which measures the force of blood when the heart is actually pumping) was significantly less forceful than that of healthy normal patients. In addition, their ejection fraction, a measurement of the heart's pumping efficiency, was unusually low.

The Italian doctors put those patients on human growth hormone for six months and, at the end of that time, not only was there a significant increase in their exercise endurance, but their indexes of cardiac function were now identical to those of the healthy control patients.[9] Apparently, growth hormone had done it again.

WHAT ARE WE WAITING FOR?

It seems to be apparent that in human growth hormone we have uncovered one of the main sources of human vitality—contributing to and improving muscle strength, cardiac function, immune function, and protection of the central nervous system. Nor is that all. Growth hormone is a jack-of-all-trades. It produces more rapid recovery after surgery, it helps burn patients recover, it reverses age-related atrophy of major organs such as the liver and the kidneys, and some doctors are now using it to treat patients with advanced emphysema. It can't cure the damaged lungs, but because of the HGH-induced increase in muscle power, the diaphragm contracts more forcefully and more air is brought into the lungs, allowing patients with late-stage lung disease to have a few more years of functional life.[10]

Does Growth Hormone Work Alone?

Perhaps this is the chief fallacy that weakens modern medicine's approach to understanding nutritional and hormonal therapies. It's clear from all that I've told you in the past two chapters that HGH is a startling therapy with a capacity to do certain things that perhaps no other hormone or drug we're aware of can do. And yet that doesn't mean it should be given in isolation, nor does it mean that it's nearly as effective alone as it is when the individual taking it is also exercising, eating well, and taking other nutrients and possibly other hormones. Despite my occasional analogies to an automobile engine that needs gas to run, the body is not a simple machine. It is an incredibly complicated whole with incredibly diverse needs.

I never treat a patient with just one substance. If he or she is receiving HGH from me, then you can be certain that that person is also receiving vitamins and minerals in abundance and almost certainly some of the other hormones discussed in this book. And advice on diet and exercise will be part of the package. Pro-longevity hormones deserve a pro-longevity lifetime health plan.

Consider Meg Bowen, a sixty-six-year-old patient under treatment with a colleague of mine. Meg has been on estrogen replacement therapy for more than a decade. I'm convinced that has helped maintain her bones and her overall physical conditioning. She looks wonderful. She says her friends tell her she looks ten years younger than her age. I don't think they're far off. Nonetheless, two years ago Meg was starting to feel the first indications of her years. Her energy was down a little bit, her hair had thinned, and in the spring and fall, pollen allergies would reduce her to misery. Then one winter she had a severe flu followed by pneumonia. That really took it out of her.

Her physician, Dr. Sam Baxis, of Key Biscayne, Florida, put her on DHEA and convinced her to try growth hormone. The changes she experienced soon afterward were dramatic. Within three months she felt a flood of energy. Her hair thickened again with better texture. The changes in her muscle strength were obvious. She started an exercise program using a treadmill and three pound weights—about half an hour a day.

And there was one other change Meg hadn't expected. She had the beginning of a cataract in her right eye. The progression of the condition not only halted, but in Ruth's opinion her eyesight improved. Assuming that it was human growth hormone that produced this effect, Ruth is not the only person to notice eye improvement after HGH replacement therapy. Dr. Julian Whitaker, a well-known physician and medical writer, reports that his own eyesight improved to such an extent after he began HGH that he seldom needs his glasses for reading anymore. There has been speculation that HGH strengthens eye muscle fibers, contributing to focus and lessening eyestrain.

Meg's reactions are simple and straightforward: "I just feel good all the time. I've got lots of energy, more than I've had in years, and I wouldn't go without growth hormone." I think that the most dramatic changes Meg Bowen has experienced are, in all probability, due to the four units of human growth hormone she's taking weekly. But I wouldn't discount the importance of everything else she's doing right. Your body appreciates every good thing you do for it. Someone like Meg who has a full anti-aging program in place and complete determination to live life to the fullest is simply two or three steps ahead of all the rest of us. If you could meet her, you'd see what I mean.

And, while I have her, let me mention one other thing you may already have noticed. For whatever reason, there are far fewer women on HGH than men. I don't know if women are reluctant to incur the expense; or if they think that a therapy that increases muscle is inherently appropriate to men; or if they're more cautious than their male counterparts about undertaking a treatment that's still controversial. But I have noticed that the women who do get growth hormone do just as well on it as men and are equally happy with the results.

SOME STUDIES ARE DESTINED TO FAIL

I couldn't do full justice to the complexities of growth hormone without mentioning a recent study (1996) published in the prestigious *Annals of Internal Medicine* and written up in some of the news media as proof of the ineffectiveness of human growth hormone as an anti-aging therapy. The study was done at the University of California, San Francisco, on fifty-two healthy older men (average age: seventy-five) who had well-preserved mental and physical abilities.[11]

The scientists gave half the patients growth hormone (approximately twelve units weekly) for six months and the other half a placebo. There were some side effects in the form of fluid retention and joint aches, which I attribute to the size of the dose. At the end of the period of study, there was little change in the untreated group. The patients on growth hormone had gained an average of 4.3 percent of lean muscle mass and had decreased their fat by 13.1 percent, but, in spite of these body-composition changes, the authors of the study reported seeing no significant improvement in mental or physical functionality. They therefore concluded that growth hormone was not a desirable therapeutic approach to address normal aging in healthy older men.

When I looked at the study, I found its conclusions unacceptable for a number of reasons. First, it hardly qualified as a true indication of what HGH can do for the average aging person. It was, in effect, an attempt to learn if the small minority of elderly men who have retained all their youthful functions at a high level could be turned into supermen simply by taking a hormone. I don't think that's possible, and I think you'll notice that most of the people whose improvements are described in this book, either had physical problems that needed improving or took active charge of their health by exercising and adding other nutrients and hormones to their bodies. I don't doubt that the subjects of the University of California study would have significantly improved their functionality, too, if, in addition to taking HGH, they had improved their diets and begun a physical fitness program. They might, indeed, have ended up as supermen for their age; instead they simply ended up with less fat and more muscle.

The other area in which the study falls short is in interpretation of the actual results. The results, after all, were very attractive. Let me summarize them. The men who got growth hormone:

- Lost an average of twenty-three pounds of fat in six months.
- Gained eight pounds of functional, protein-based lean tissue.
- Gained one and three-fourths pounds of bone mineral (calcium).
- Gained 3 percent in knee strength.
- Gained 12 percent in skin thickness.
- Gained 12 percent in a mental dexterity test.

I think it is dubious to claim that these results—achieved by sitting on one's duff—are simply nothing. And the last item on that list is very interesting. The authors of the study actually conducted several mental function tests on their subjects. The test that was interesting was one that measured visual tracking skills, hand-eye coordination, and concentration, and it was this test that showed the highly significant 12 percent gain. The other tests involve such things as knowing what year it is or what day of the week and are really only useful in people showing significant mental decline. Naturally, the subjects of this study did equally well on such tests both before and after they took HGH, but when the absence of improvement in these tests was averaged in with the more complex test on which there was a 12 percent gain, the final score failed to achieve statistical significance. It strikes me that this is a poorly designed method of measuring changes in mental function.

In any event, if this is the study that disproves the efficacy of HGH in the elderly—and it has been touted as such—then those who oppose hormone therapy had better go back to the drawing boards. They will need a heftier club than this.

SAILING ON

My conclusions remain unremittingly positive. In thirty years of practicing medicine, I haven't seen a new therapeutic tool come along with anything like such power over such a range of human ailments. Nor have I in that time seen anything that so dramatically affects the simple quality of life of patients who don't have anything fundamentally out of whack except the age they've reached and the way it makes them feel.

Perhaps a growth-hormone patient named Oliver Madan described the feeling HGH gives older people best of all.

Oliver's seventy-seven, and he didn't have much wrong with him except the fact that he was really starting to feel his age. No energy; no get-up-and-go; no muscles; falling asleep all the time, even when he was driving his car. Oliver's conclusion: his life was winding down.

After eight months of HGH, he came to a different conclusion. Now he no longer needs so much sleep—and certainly not while driving. Now the muscles in his legs and his arms are hardening. Now he runs up the steps in his house "as if I were twenty years younger."

"I thought my life was almost over," Oliver told me. "But now I'm planning to go on to a hundred."

CHAPTER FIVE

Growth Hormone: What If You Plan to Take It?

I KNOW A DOCTOR IN TEXAS WHO RECENTLY DECIDED TO TREAT his ninety-five-year-old mother with HGH. Over the previous year she had grown exceedingly weak and despondent and had finally become bedridden. The doctor couldn't find any precise constitutional reason for her state; she simply didn't seem to have the strength to live anymore. Within two months of taking HGH, his mom was walking again. Within three months she was happy to be alive. If the illness that doctor was treating wasn't aging, I don't know what to call it.

This is interesting because, certain as I am that human growth hormone will be increasingly used in coming decades to treat such medical conditions as heart disease and Alzheimer's, I'm well aware that its use in the control of aging is another matter.

Our own Food and Drug Administration is very specific about the fact that it does not regard aging as an illness. A reasonable view to them, no doubt, even if many gerontologists tend toward the opposite opinion and speak of aging as the ultimate illness. Unfortunately in such disputes there is a good deal more at stake than verbal hairsplitting. The FDA's choice of a definition is done with a purpose. If aging is no illness, then clearly any medicine created for the purpose of slowing or reversing aging is not medically sound and not appropriate for government approval. And drug companies are well aware of this. They know that if they wish to have a drug approved, they must demonstrate its effectiveness against a "real" illness. Even when applying for approval to treat a real illness such as Alzheimer's, arthritis, or Parkinson's, aging need not—and should not—be mentioned in their submission to the FDA.

Thus the development of HGH as an anti-aging therapy is going to be left largely to the initiative of doctors and patients. That is what's occurring, still slowly but more and more noticeably, nationwide. This fundamentally unusual and significantly unregulated situation is advantageous in one sense. As soon as the price goes down, the use of growth hormone to reverse and slow aging is going to proceed with an astonishing speed that would never occur in the normal development of a significant new medical treatment. The same situation is disadvantageous in that quicker development implies less testing to determine side effects and hazards. And clearly nothing as potent as human growth hormone can be entirely without risk.

In this chapter I intend to look first at the risks involved in low-dose administration of HGH. Then we'll consider who's making growth hormone, how it's being made, how reliable the suppliers are, how it's being brought into this country, and how you'll go about getting it, should you and your physician decide this is the therapy for you. Finally, we'll take a peek into the future.

THE PRUDENT APPROACH

I have two strong opinions about growth hormone, which I hold with equal vehemence. One is that restoration of youthful levels of HGH is potentially the most powerful and beneficial aid to a vital long life that the human race has ever discovered. The other is that this is not a substance that an individual man or woman should even consider taking independantly of a physician's advice and guidance.

It is true that the relative infrequency of side effects caused by growth hormone is genuinely reassuring; it can only be explained by the fact that HGH is a natural product of our own endocrine glands and safe and prudent treatment involves simply restoring it to the levels that were present and well tolerated in young adulthood. That this is the true explanation for its impressive safety record receives support from the fact that almost all recorded adverse effects have occurred when the hormone is given at doses significantly higher than what the human body normally produces in its youthful prime.

In giving hormones it has become increasingly clear that we are wise to follow nature. In medicine this is called giving physiological doses—amounts that the body naturally produces. The opposite approach is to give pharmacological doses—amounts in excess of what any healthy human body would produce for itself. Unless a strong series of medical studies eventually shows that some compelling advantage can be had from such an approach, I definitely advise against pharmacological doses of HGH.

The Range of Side Effects

Now let's look at every conceivable side effect that the several dozen growth hormone studies conducted so far have identified.

First off, I would like to mention, only in order to dismiss, one grotesque and fearful side effect of overdosage. In the early days of giving HGH, there was some apprehension that acromegaly might result. Acromegaly is a rare disease of giantism or abnormal bone growth that occurs when the pituitary gland secretes greatly excessive levels of growth hormone over a long period. It usually results from a benign tumor on the pituitary gland. A childhood occurrence of acromegaly causes giantism, as in the case of Robert Wadlow, the tallest documented human, who reached eight feet eleven inches before his early death. In cases where the excessive secretion of growth hormone occurs after adulthood, increase in overall body size occurs somewhat differently. There is only limited growth in the bones of the extremities and of the face (causing facial deformity). Fortunately, acromegaly has never occurred in a planned program of growth hormone replacement, even at doses far higher than I would recommend.

The side effects that do occasionally occur are these:

- edema (water retention)
- carpal tunnel syndrome
- hypertension
- increased blood glucose levels

When growth hormone is supplemented at too high a level, these are, indeed, very natural consequences of its action. Consider edema. It is a basic medical maxim that body water content decreases with age. Tissues become slightly desiccated. In fact, by the time young men and women become senior citizens, the percentage of water by weight in their bodies has declined by 10 percent. When HGH levels are brought up, tissue water content is restored to a younger level. I have not seen significant edema in any of my own growth hormone patients, although I do notice that skin texture improves with more normal hydration.

The important point to note is that when a sudden increase in HGH has resulted in symptomatic edema, this has only occurred when patients were given doses higher than the body would naturally produce. In the early studies on growth hormone, the doctors conducting the experiments were not at all certain what a normal dose would be. Even Daniel Rudman, in his famous 1990 study of HGH administered to elderly men, used sixteen units of HGH weekly. That's approximately four times the amount needed to bring substantial improvement in the average sixty-five-year-old. In other words, I and most physicians using HGH supplementation today seldom prescribe more than four units a week. As it happened, none of Rudman's patients suffered significant edema (although there was one rather serious case of carpal tunnel syndrome). But in certain other experimental studies conducted at even higher dosages, edema has been a problem. If you look at the dosages in Table 5.1, you'll see the levels of supplementation used in eleven well-regarded studies of human growth hormone. At the higher doses, some edema was noted.

My advice to patients is first, of course, to supplement at a safe physiological dose, which is usually four units per week. When a patient already has a problem with water retention, I watch his or her progress more closely. So far, problems have not occurred. If they did, I would naturally lower the dose or stop for a while, and then follow the patient closely to see if the problem gradually abated. I believe that in most cases this would occur, as the body adjusted to its new level of HGH. Patients who required diuretics (water pills) before beginning HGH will need to continue on them afterward.

Any significant increase in fluid retention raises blood pressure, and this is undoubtedly the reason why hypertensive patients have experienced blood pressure increases in some studies of the hormone. Nevertheless, if a person's hypertension is being controlled by diet or medication, I do not regard high blood pressure as a reason for not enjoying all the other major health advantages supplied by HGH.

Table 5.1
Dosages in Eleven Major Studies of
Human Growth Hormone

Author	Year	Dose (in units per week)
Crist	1987	12
Beshyan	1994	15
Rudman	1990	16
Bengt-ake	1993	18
Whitehead	1992	28
Cuneo	1991	30
Salamon	1989	30
Skaggs	1991	34–62
Richelson	1994	35
Kaiser	1991	100
Orme	1992	122

Once again, problems do not appear to arise when a person is taking a physiological dose—four units per week—and wisdom counsels close consultation with a physician.

Carpal Tunnel Syndrome

The side effect most commonly seen in studies using large doses of human growth hormone is carpal tunnel syndrome. The carpal tunnel is a channel under the ligament crossing the front of your wrist through which major nerves pass to your hand. Pressure on those nerves can cause numbness, tingling, or weakness in the hand. This is a fairly common syndrome, especially in middle age and especially in women, not infrequently among people who spend a good deal of time working at a typewriter or computer keyboard and who suffer the effects of what has been dubbed repetitive motion injury. The effects can be fairly painful and unpleasant. Supplemental vitamins, especially B_6 (pyridoxine), will often help or prevent this condition. Vitamin deficiency may be a cause.

Increases in levels of growth hormone speed tissue repair and protein synthesis in the body. This can create a greater demand for all nutrients, which may therefore aggravate any preexisting vitamin deficiency. If one adds to this two other effects that HGH may cause, namely increase in body water content and slight increases in the bone mass of the forearm and wrist, it's easy to see that HGH could precipitate carpal tunnel syndrome if it was on the verge of occurring anyway. Both those effects, incidentally—increased hydration and stronger bones—are beneficial to the body as a whole.

I believe from my own experience and that of others that an aggravation or sudden onset of carpal tunnel syndrome after the commencement of growth hormone supplementation is going to be rare or nonexistent at the doses we currently use for anti-aging. Your physician should be aware of the possibility, however, and, if you already have a tendency toward carpal tunnel syndrome, he or she should take you into a supplement program that includes a spectrum of vitamins, minerals, and trace elements, including an insurance dose of B_6.

It is important to also consider overall nutritional status. As tissue repair, healing, and cell replacement are speeded up by growth hormone replacement, the need for nutrients of all types also increases. Protein intake must be adequate to build up new tissues. Vitamins, minerals, and trace elements are all utilized in higher amounts as the metabolic rate increases and cells are replaced and repaired. If the body is deficient or borderline in essential nutrients, an increase in cell growth can aggravate or create deficiencies that might not have been apparent otherwise. It is certainly wise to seek out a physician skilled in clinical nutrition and preventive medicine to help you manage your use of growth hormone therapy. In Chapters Thirteen and Fourteen, I'll outline a typical program of diet and nutritional supplementation to go along with anti-aging hormones.

If you can improve your nutritional status as you begin hormonal replacement therapy, you will be far likelier to receive significant benefits and be better protected against side effects. I have observed that regular exercise, even just a brisk walk several times per week, will also increase benefits.

Risky for Diabetics?

Once again the major consideration seems to be dosage. Growth hormone—supplemented in amounts considerably higher than necessary for reaching a young person's levels—has been shown to raise blood-sugar levels by antagonizing insulin. But in normal clinical practice, my own and that of many other physicians, increases in blood-sugar levels are miniscule to nonexistent. From a practical point of view therefore, growth hormone replacement ought to pose no sort of threat to people with diabetes or borderline diabetes. As with all administration of growth hormone, it is essential that individuals consult their physicians, undergo lab tests, and conform their anti-aging health plans to the requirements of their bodies.

THE SOURCES OF HUMAN GROWTH HORMONE

Where does human growth hormone—the kind we inject—come from? Who makes it, who wants to sell it, who's allowed to sell it, and—the bottom line—how can you obtain a safe and reliable supply if you eventually decide that it will be a part of your personal anti-aging regimen?

What About Cancer?

Since growth hormone stimulates the growth of many different sorts of tissues, there has been speculation that it might increase the risk of cancer. All the evidence so far would indicate that HGH is not a risk factor. One published report of growth hormone research stated that in 16,604 person-years of treatment—a person-year is one person receiving a therapy for one year—there was no increase in the reported levels of cancer.

An even more convincing indicator that cancer risk from HGH is low, if it exists at all, is the overall experience of growth hormone administration to growth-deficient children over the course of the past twenty years. During this period tens of thousands of children have received the hormone for periods as long as ten consecutive years. Recent reviews have shown that the incidence of leukemia and lymphoma, the most common pediatric malignancies, did not increase.[1]

A smaller study was done in England on young brain-tumor patients.[2] Because the radiation given in brain cancer therapy often damages the pituitary gland, a significant percentage of these patients are supplemented with growth hormone in the years following their treatment. The records kept by the British physicians showed that among 207 young brain-tumor patients, the individuals who later received growth hormone did not have any higher rate of tumor recurrence than those who did not receive HGH.

As of this time, the evidence indicates that HGH does not increase the risk of cancer and does not cause established cancers to grow more rapidly.

These are important questions and deserve serious discussion not only for their own sakes but because they relate to the chief drawback of HGH: its monstrous expense. Depending upon the dose that an elderly patient and his or her doctor decide to administer, the cost will usually be somewhere between $8,000 and $16,000 a year or approximately $160 to $320 a week. Certainly a good bit more than the price of dinner at a good restaurant on a Saturday night. And regrettably, far beyond the means of most people who have a grave and genuine need for growth hormone therapy.

The main reason for this exorbitant price is competition—or, in this case, the lack of it. Up until now two companies have maintained a monopoly on HGH in the American market, even though there are four other reputable companies in Europe who make the substance and are eager to import it. It appears that the monopoly is about to crack. In the next few years the price is almost certainly going to begin tumbling down, and then, willynilly, whether our government's bureaucracies like it or not, a new age of anti-aging medicine is going to be upon us.

Up until now, growth hormone has remained tightly restricted in the United States because various forms of exclusivity have worked in conjunction with the wishes of the FDA. Although, as a natural substance, growth hormone would appear immune to patenting, in practice, things worked out differently. Genentech, a large biotechnology corporation in the San Francisco Bay area, developed four key patents in the 1980s protecting the processes and procedures whereby HGH is manufactured. Genentech's process involves giant culture vats filled with *E. coli* bacteria—yes, that's the same bacteria naturally found in your body. Recombinant DNA technology allows these bacterial cultures to produce natural growth hormone.

The actual process of making the growth hormone molecule itself is no longer a terribly difficult one, now that the code sequence has been worked out for the human gene that causes the pituitary gland to string together growth hormone's 191-amino-acid chain. The gene, once made, is transplanted into an *E. coli* bacteria, which is then allowed to grow and multiply in a nutrient broth at approximately body temperature. After the *E. coli* has grown and multiplied sufficiently, a purification process is done to separate out the growth hormone. This is currently the most difficult and sophisticated portion of the manufacturing process. Without very gentle and delicate handling, many growth hormone molecules will be damaged. Growth hormone is not simply one long chain of amino acids—it is folded and twisted in a precise manner, with its branches connected at very specific points in cross-linkages.

Hormones work by precisely fitting into receptors on the surface of cells and cell membranes. The process is very similar to fitting a key into a lock. All of the little twists, turns, and grooves on a key must be exactly right or the key will not open the lock. In the same way, the exact three-dimensional configuration of growth hormone must precisely fit into cell receptors or there will be no growth hormone activity. If purification and packaging of HGH is properly done, the molecule retains its shape and will do its job.

Genentech created procedures that successfully dealt with these problems and that ensured that the final product would be exactly like pure growth hormone. In the 1980s Eli Lilly, the pharmaceutical giant, tried to make the hormone using somewhat similar procedures, and Genentech sued for patent violations. After some fierce legal tussles in the federal courts in Indianapolis, the smaller but feisty biotechnology company agreed to license its process patents to Lilly in return for approximately $145 million. At that stage, both companies had approval from the Food and Drug Administration to market the hormone for pituitary deficiencies in children. And, indeed, their exclusive marketing control was not only protected by Genentech's patents but by the fact that the FDA had declared HGH an "orphan drug" and under the law granted the two companies the exclusive right for several years to be the only ones making marketing claims regarding HGH's effectiveness against growth deficiency in children. There seems to have been an unwritten understanding with the FDA that neither company would allow their growth hormone to be used for any other purpose.

However, in 1995 orphan drug exclusivity for marketing claims ran out, and several European firms poised themselves for entry. Two of the firms, Novo Nordisk, a Scandinavian biotechnology giant, and Biotechnology General, which manufactures in Israel, make HGH by an *E. coli* bacterial process similar to Genentech's. Both companies maintain, however, that their processes are sufficiently different that Genentech's patents do not apply. Genentech first filed a complaint with the International Trade Commission claiming patent violation. The suit was thrown out because the presiding judge ruled Genentech was withholding important documents relevant to the case. Novo Nordisk and Biotechnology General promptly started procedures to import HGH, and Genentech just as promptly filed a new suit against them in federal court, the Southern District Court in New York City, where the battle goes on to this day.

Happily for all of us who would like to see the price of the hormone go down, the other two European firms seem to be protected from legal challenges by Genentech.

Ares Sorono, headquartered in Switzerland, uses mammalian cells instead of *E. coli* bacteria as the basis of its manufacturing process and therefore is free of any patent competition with Genentech. Consequently they can enter the American market at any time with FDA approval, and they have applied for that. It has been reported that they're building a new plant in the United States, where they intend to manufacture growth hormone.

In a very interesting further development, Ares Sorono has done some very sound scientific research on the use of HGH to treat advanced AIDS patients suffering with cachexia (massive weight loss and muscle wasting). The results of that research were very positive, and apparently they expect to receive FDA approval to market growth hormone for that indication. Such a step would undoubtedly have a profound impact on the prospects for expanded use of human growth hormone. The muscle wasting that takes place with AIDS has a certain similarity to the muscle wasting of age, and, of course, HGH reverses both forms of wasting by similar means. I can only assume that the publicity HGH would receive—assisted as it would be by the advocacy of the gay community—might well combine with the breaking of Genentech's and Lilly's monopoly hold to loosen restrictions on the hormone's use.

Another company, which has entered the market through Mexico is Pharmacia AB, located in Stockholm, Sweden, but it has been difficult to obtain reliable information on the quality of their product.

Another growth hormone manufacturer has not yet attempted to enter the U.S. market but would clearly like to. BIOFA AB is a Lithuanian company that before the collapse of the Soviet Union was an important manufacturer of recombinant DNA products in the Soviet bloc. Within the last year, BIOFA has privatized and has thus far received the equivalent of our FDA approval in a number of other countries. BIOFA need not fear patent disputes with Genentech because they have produced a form of growth hormone that does not infringe on Genentech's patents.

Nature's own growth hormone has a 191-amino-acid sequence. BIOFA has taken advantage of the fact that only the front end, so to speak, of the molecule fits into cellular receptor sites. To understand this better, picture a key fitting into a lock. The front part of the key that actually turns the tumblers must be made with absolute precision, but the handle can be square or round or oval or solid or hollow or holed. It turns out that at the nitrogen end of the amino acid sequence—what we might call the back end of the growth hormone molecule or the handle on the key— very tiny changes to the sequence have no functional significance. Consequently BIOFA produces a 190-amino-acid sequence in their form of growth hormone, which bypasses Genentech's patents. This may be a case of the San Francisco company being hoisted with its own petard. It has been reported that in the 1980s, hoping to circumnavigate a University of California patent, Genentech added an extra amino acid molecule at the same position to produce a 192-amino-acid sequence. This would make it somewhat difficult for them to argue the unfairness of the Lithuanian company's move. HGH with one amino acid more or less at the inactive end of the hormone structure has been proven conclusively in clinical trials to be identical in its action. The FDA approved Genentech's earlier version, which is good evidence for its safety and effectiveness.

As demand expands, other biotechnology companies around the world will undoubtedly begin to manufacture HGH. I have heard that China may be preparing to enter the market in Asia.

As a physician my only interest is in seeing the cost of growth hormone go down while the high quality that currently exists is maintained. But it's probably time for us to consider the question of quality while describing the normal procedures for obtaining growth hormone that an older person must currently follow.

Usually, It's Through Mexico

Many individuals who want to take human growth hormone to counter the effects of aging hesitate to do so because they assume that the FDA's attempts to restrict its use to growth-deficient children means that they and their physician will be involved in some sort of illegality if they use it for other purposes. That is absolutely not the case. It is a well-established legal principle in American medicine that a physician may use any approved drug for therapeutic purposes other than those for which it was designed, if that physician feels such a use is best for his patient. This is called "off-label" use and is, in fact, quite common. In spite of the FDA's successful attempts to coerce Genentech and Lilly into restricting sales of growth hormone purely for use in the treatment of growth deficiency and dwarfism in children, the "off-label" principle still applies, and, if a supply of the growth hormone can be obtained, the doctor and his patient are perfectly within their rights in using it.

The question, of course, is how to obtain that supply.

As we've noted, Genentech and Lilly, the only two companies currently permitted to sell HGH in the United States, sell growth hormone solely to physicians and organizations that can demonstrate patient by patient, through the use of growth charts and other data, that use of the hormone is restricted to its "FDA-approved" uses. Therefore, the thousands of older patients who are currently using growth hormone must be getting it elsewhere, and they are.

Most of it is coming from Europe through Mexico. However, the hormone is on the FDA's "hot list," and people who try to import large supplies of HGH across the border to sell in this country are stopped by U.S. Customs inspectors at the point of entry into the United States.

This does not apply to small amounts (three months' supply or less) for personal use. If you can show a doctor's prescription, you will not be bothered if you bring your own medicine across the border. But if you're among the many people who don't find it convenient to go to Mexico or Europe four times a year, then you will need to find a reliable supplier in this country, who has established his own method of access to overseas sources. Which is literally what he should be bringing you. No growth hormone is manufactured in Mexico, although almost all of it used in the U.S. for anti-aging purposes passes through that most porous of border countries.

Your supplier is most likely to be a physician whom you trust or a reputable compounding pharmacy. (Several possible sources are listed in Appendix Three.) Women's International Pharmacy in Sun City West, Arizona, phone 1-800-699-8143, is my preferred supplier.

In spite of the FDA's interest in keeping growth hormone under wraps, if your physician thinks HGH is safe and appropriate for you, there's no legal problem in taking it. A compounding pharmacy merely needs to receive a written prescription from your doctor and then fill that prescription and provide you with your growth hormone. Compounding pharmacies are an important aspect of our medical freedom. Most ordinary pharmacies simply count out ready-made pills and capsules from a large bottle into an individual prescription bottle for personal use.

A compounding pharmacist will prepare whatever medicine a licensed physician regards as therapeutically desirable, or, as is the case with growth hormone, will take steps to obtain it. Indeed, if you had a physician unusual enough to decide that ground-up bat's wing or rhinoceros horn was just the thing for you, it would (theoretically, at least) be quite legal for a compounding pharmacist to provide them. FDA approval is not an issue with compounding pharmacies.

You should take note of what brand of growth hormone is being provided for your use, and the vials of growth hormone should have the original labels of the manufacturer. If you have any doubt about the source of the growth hormone, ask the pharmacy if they can provide you with a certificate of analysis conducted by a qualified laboratory that shows acceptable purity. Some physicians do their own quality control investigations and dispense the HGH directly to patients from their offices.

There have been reported instances of growth hormone being diluted in Mexico and then sold in the United States. I recently received reports of a growth hormone product that came in through Mexico with a German company named on the label. Mexican authorities I have talked to tell me that they have determined that the German company does not exist, and the product actually comes from Pakistan. Whether or not it contains any growth hormone is in doubt at this time.

Until a wider distribution of growth hormone in the United States makes it easier to acquire, finding a physician you can trust and/or a reliable compounding pharmacist is your best assurance that you will not be cheated.

Stability

When you receive a supply of growth hormone, you will want to keep it refrigerated. The hormone is shipped and sold in a freeze-dried form sealed in a sterile vial, to which a weak salt solution is added when it is prepared for injection. As long as it is kept in its freeze-dried form at a temperature of approximately 34 to 38 degrees Fahrenheit, it will remain stable for up to eighteen months. Even at room temperature, the freeze-dried form will retain its potency for about a month or longer. However, once water is added to it, it should be used within two weeks if refrigerated and within two or three days if unrefrigerated. It should never be allowed to become warmer than 80 degrees Fahrenheit or it will more rapidly lose its potency.

It's important to keep growth hormone free of any contaminants, especially once it's in its liquid form. Use a new syringe every time you inject yourself—otherwise any contamination on the needle of the used syringe may get into the vial carrying contaminants. Blood residues on a used needle may also contain proteolytic enzymes that can begin to digest the remaining growth hormone in the vial and cause bacteria to multiply inside the vial.

MORE RESEARCH IS IN THE WORKS

Growth hormone is going to remain in the news because the reverberations of Daniel Rudman's original clinical trial have certainly not died down. Under the sponsorship of the National Institute on Aging, nine new studies on the effects of growth hormone administration to the elderly are being conducted at institutions as prestigious as Johns Hopkins School of Medicine and Stanford University Medical Center. Each study is different, but some of the areas being investigated include HGH's effects on cardiovascular function, on aerobic capacity, on bone density (a treatment for osteoporosis), and on mental function. The first published results will probably appear in 1997.

CHAPTER SIX

DHEA: Super Hormone in Search of Its Identity

"If you want to maintain a youthful level of health, then you have to be youthful physiologically. You have to maintain youthful levels of these hormones."

—WILLIAM REGELSON, M.D.

AT SIXTY-SEVEN, AMY WOOLF FOUND THAT EVEN GETTING OUT of bed in the morning took almost as much energy as she had. "I've gotten used to feeling bad," she told me. "It becomes a way of life." Amy, a mild diabetic, was so tired that I considered diagnosing her condition as Chronic Fatigue Syndrome. But, when I tried her out on DHEA, in less than thirty days she came back and told me, "I've never had so much energy in my life. I feel like I'm twenty-five again." That was three or four years ago, pretty early in my career as a doctor who prescribes hormones. I was amazed then; nowadays I hear similar stories from men and women and am not surprised.

Growth hormone certainly has the most obvious and visible effects on the human body, but it may turn out to be DHEA that is the more interesting of the pro-longevity hormones, primarily because of its ready availability, low cost, and absence of significant side effects at replacement doses. It has the advantage of being good, to a greater or lesser extent, for almost everything. A claim like that ought to arouse your skepticism. When it comes to dehydroepiandrosterone—that's its full, formal, chemical, tongue-twisting title—a look into the medical literature tends to defuse skepticism rather quickly.

I expect that not many of you will have heard of this hormone, and I know for a fact that few doctors have given it a thought since the days when they read a paragraph or two about it in Basic Endocrinology. Yet our adrenal glands produce more DHEA than all the other adrenal hormones combined. If it doesn't have a profound significance, then your body is guilty of profligate excess in its secretion. Which is inherently unlikely, for the human body runs a tight ship.

Our only problem has been figuring out what vital purposes this important hormone serves.

We do find that when people take it, they feel emphatically *younger*. Ask Joan Baldick, one of the participants in a University of California study. For six months she took a DHEA pill not knowing whether it was the real thing or a placebo. But: "My body knew. I slept less, but I slept better. I felt eager to get out of bed in the morning. And there's no question I felt more feminine, more sensuous. I sure did notice the difference."

If DHEA makes a difference it's not surprising, for some researchers call it "the most reliable biomarker of aging," and certainly from a lab technician's point of view, it's a superb measuring rod of age. At twenty, you have extraordinary quantities of DHEA in your body. By the age of eighty, you have about 10 percent of that original abundance. And during the intervening six decades, the graph of loss will be a steady declining line with very little in the way of eccentric bumps or dips. Is this coincidental or do youth and vigor go down as DHEA goes down—perhaps, to a significant extent, *because* DHEA goes down?

Since DHEA can be readily converted into other hormones, including cortisone, progesterone, estrogen, and testosterone, scientists originally thought this richly supplied adrenal hormone was simply a transition substance, a reservoir upon which the body could draw when it needed to manufacture other steroids. Further research demonstrated, however, that most cells in the body contain specific DHEA receptors, the sole function of which is to bind DHEA. This is as clear an indication as we can get that DHEA has essential functions of its own in the human body.

What are those functions? We're going to speculate as the chapter continues, but I'll tell you now, we won't reach any hard and fast conclusions. DHEA is still a thorny biomedical enigma. But if the precise mechanisms of its action remain elusive, its ultimate effects are crystal clear.

We now know that low levels of DHEA are strongly associated with heart attack risk. We have abundant evidence that high levels of DHEA protect against cancer. We've found that it helps in treating and preventing diabetes. We've seen in animal studies and in double blind studies on humans that it aids memory, eases depression, and causes a striking improvement in an individual's sense of psychological and physical well-being. Finally, we know that it so strongly supports the immune system that many scientists have become convinced that a shortage of this very hormone contributes significantly to the immune system's collapse in old age. If this were not sufficient, there is also evidence that DHEA can help in the treatment of osteoporosis, rheumatoid arthritis, obesity, and chronic fatigue. It mediates stress, improves sleep, and appears to ginger up the sex drive in some folks.

Perhaps, after all, the body knows what it's doing when it provides the vigorous and active twenty-year-old with copious quantities of DHEA.

FIXING WHAT AILS YOU? SOMETIMES IT SEEMS THAT WAY

We can all see that, on the face of it, DHEA is a model pro-longevity hormone. It is a normal part of our metabolism, something the body produces daily. Yet it becomes radically depleted as we grow older. Most important of all, when it is replaced, the body accepts that replacement and shows emphatically positive effects.

I started giving DHEA to my patients five years ago, using it cautiously, in limited amounts. I made careful laboratory measurements of their blood levels to ensure that what I gave them brought them only up to what was normal in a healthy young adult. The response was pretty striking. Men and women who had noticed they were slipping and sliding into age, into a place they didn't want to be yet, came back to my office two or three weeks later and said, *whatever you do for me, please don't stop giving me DHEA.*

Some were people who had absolutely nothing wrong with them. George Bloom was only forty-one years old, but his blood level of DHEAS (the form in which the hormone is measured) was low for his age. George is a take-vitamins-and-exercise sort of person, determined to slow the aging process before it even begins. He asked me for DHEA, and I prescribed it in appropriate doses. After a few months on the hormone, he noticed that his energy level was markedly higher, his skin was thicker and moister, and he was sleeping six and a half hours a night instead of eight and waking rested. George says he feels six or seven years younger, and, as he puts it, "When you're on DHEA, it feels as if every cell in your body is just humming." That's a common observation of people taking this pro-longevity hormone. George has also noticed that his sex drive has ratcheted sharply upward.

Carol Constance was forty-seven, and she had more immediate reasons for replacing hormones. I suppose it would be fair to say Carol was going through a pretty serious mid-life crisis with everything hitting at once. Her menstrual cycle had been going haywire for about a year. Each month she had terrible migraines around the time of her period. And for her that was really twice a month since her cycle now went for only ten to fifteen days. It was winter, and Carol was suffering terrible depression. As she told me, "I kept thinking of my wasted life, of all the things I thought I would do when I was nineteen that I'd never done. I would lie in bed and wail during the night."

If Carol needed more problems, asthma provided them. It had surfaced in her life in 1988, and by 1995 it had gotten markedly worse. Carol slept with her cats, and I told her she really shouldn't. She told me bluntly that as she was now divorced, she certainly wasn't going to kick her cats out of bed.

And then DHEA came on the scene, and, to my astonishment and hers, somewhat miraculously, almost everything turned around.

> Within an hour after taking my first capsule, I suddenly found I could breathe again. That month my periods went back to normal—I was on my old regular twenty-seven-day cycle—and my headaches disappeared. My depression lifted within the first few days. Two months after I started DHEA I joined a dance class. It had always been a childhood dream to dance. I feel like a teenager, as if I were renewing myself.

It has been over a year since Carol Constance went on DHEA. She's had one or two very minor asthma attacks in that time, but not a trace of her other problems. The only side effect she's noticed has been an occasional outbreak of acne, which went away as soon as she interrupted her DHEA for a few days. I've found that acne only occurs in patients who are quite clearly deficient in DHEA, as Carol was. The problem soon disappears after normal levels are reached, apparently an adjustment of the oil glands in the skin to the restoration of youthful quantities of DHEA.

George and Carol's results are typical of the wide range of apparently unconnected positive effects that this powerful adrenal hormone produces in the human body. Therefore is it surprising that scientific studies have shown a real statistical relationship between how much DHEA you have at any given age and how healthy you are? We've all seen people who at fifty, sixty, or seventy-five still seem to possess what other folks have lost. In a word: Youth. I think as more research is done, we're going to find that most of these lucky individuals have more of the juice of life in their hormonal tanks than the rest of us.

Your Basic Feel-Good Hormone

The folks at the University of California have been among the most vigorous investigators of DHEA. In 1994 Samuel Yen, M.D., the head of one team on the La Jolla campus, published a double-blind study on healthy people that was charming in its simplicity. Thirteen men and seventeen women ranging in age from forty to seventy were given a "replacement dose" of DHEA—enough to bring the body's levels to the level of a vigorous young adult—for three months and a fake pill (placebo) for another three. No one knew who was receiving which until a code was broken at the study's end.

Since the thirty subjects were all healthy, there was never any question of curing illness. What happened, however—measured by answers to lengthy questionnaires—was startling enough. An overwhelming majority (67 percent of the men and 84 percent of the women) reported a "remarkable increase in perceived physical and psychological well-being" during the period in which they were on DHEA.[1]

My own experience with patients has shown over and over how frequently they come back after taking DHEA for a while and tell me—in vague but glowing terms—that their life has somehow just improved. This is an interesting response, certainly different from conventional methods of measuring physical well-being (not to mention actuarial life expectancy.)

By contrast, let's say your cholesterol level is found to be low. That suggests a decreased statistical probability of suffering a heart attack—which is certainly very fine. However, it isn't something that you can feel or sense as a part of day-to-day living. The actual perception of increased vitality that patients report when they take DHEA may seem modest in health terms. But it indicates to me that, when one supplements with the hormones that youth has abundantly, a certain reversal to youthfulness is part of the package.

A few of the conditions I haven't mentioned yet that have been reported to improve when DHEA is administered include allergies, Alzheimer's, arthritis, chemical sensitivities, chronic fatigue, elevated cholesterol, Epstein-Barr syndrome, herpes, liver disorders, lupus, menopause, recurrent infections, and senility.

The Difference Between Life and Death?

DHEA is clearly good for the healthy as well as the ill. As I look at the tremendous body of research that's been done on this adrenal hormone over the past ten or fifteen years, it has occurred to me that what it certainly seems to be doing for healthy folks is preventing them from getting sick.

Among well-conducted scientific studies in this area, the eye-opener came in 1986, when Elizabeth Barrett-

Connor, M.D., head of epidemiology at the University of California at San Diego, published a report that tracked heart attacks and deaths over a twelve-year period in 242 men aged fifty to seventy-nine. In this group, men with higher DHEA levels had a 36 percent reduction in mortality from all causes and a 48 percent reduction in mortality from heart disease.[2]

The heart disease reduction was particularly striking being so specific to one illness, and it's particularly interesting because of some confirming animal studies that have been done since. Animal studies have had singular importance in DHEA research because of a basic fact of economics. DHEA is a natural substance, unpatentable and unprofitable. Research has to be done the cheap way—on animals. No drug company will spend tens of millions of dollars conducting major clinical trials on humans. But animal research can be very suggestive.

There is a breed of rabbit called the New Zealand White that has been used in cardiovascular research since 1914. It inherits the trait of abnormally high cholesterol levels and consequently tends to rapidly form arterial plaque and die of narrowing of the arteries. Scientists at Johns Hopkins took twenty of these New Zealand Whites and using catheters caused slight irritations to the intima (the innermost lining) of the aorta in order to even further promote plaque formation. Some of the rabbits then received DHEA in their chow over the next three months, while the rest did not. In those receiving DHEA, there was an almost 50 percent reduction in plaque size, and the degree of protection was directly related to the final blood level of DHEA achieved.[3]

That study was conducted in 1988. In 1993 scientists at the Medical College of Virginia tried another variation on high-cholesterol rabbits. Both in humans and in rabbits, heart transplantation tends to cause a dangerously accelerated rate of atherosclerosis in the coronary arteries. John

Nestler, M.D., and his associates did heart transplants on forty-five rabbits and then using light microscopy observed the progressive development of arterial narrowing in these hearts. When DHEA was administered on a regular basis to these rabbits, there was a 45 percent reduction in the number of significantly narrowed vessels.[4]

Will what works in rabbits work in humans? Barrett-Connor's original study at the University of California would tend to make me believe so.

Stress and Your Aging Immune System

I wonder if the most powerful benefit of DHEA isn't going to turn out to be immune enhancement. You've already seen in the growth hormone chapters the importance that I place on this issue. Failure of immune function is what tends to kill you as you get older. The benefits of hormones can perhaps somewhat simplistically be divided into two parts. There are the benefits that make life in an aging body more pleasant, more fulfilling, more like what we enjoyed in youth. And then there are the benefits that actually extend longevity.

I believe that most of the longevity benefits of the pro-longevity hormone team will ultimately turn out to revolve around immune enhancement. If you live to be 120, it will be largely because your immune system demonstrates a superb capacity to deal with the insults of daily living.

One of those insults—both mental and physical—is the inability to adapt in healthy ways to excessive stress. Beginning in the 1930s, scientists like Dr. Hans Selye started looking at just what stress does to us. I don't know if they were surprised, but they found that stress dramatically alters the kinds and quantities of hormones released by our bodies. One of the hormones that decreases rapidly under stress is DHEA. Others increase. The hypothalamus responds to stress by secreting a substance called corticotrophin releasing factor. This, in turn, signals the pituitary gland to produce a substance that instructs the adrenals to produce corticosteroids.

The corticosteroids suppress the immune system—which is why doctors often prescribe these powerful drugs (cortisone is a well known example) to the folks who are suffering from autoimmune diseases like rheumatoid arthritis, in which the body's immune system attacks itself.

It's a well-attested fact that older people have particular problems adapting to stress. According to Dr. William Regelson of the Medical College of Virginia, older people's stress hormones rise to a higher level than young people's and remain there far longer. They are truly "stressed out," and the effect on their immune system is devastating.

It appears that one principal reason is their low levels of DHEA. In fact, many scientists now believe that one of the most important functions of DHEA is to act as a buffer hormone, a sort of normalizing hormone that deexcites and controls the activities of other hormones and enzymes in the body. This inhibitory function may explain DHEA's usefullness in controlling cancer, diabetes, and, to a certain extent, obesity. Specifically, with regard to stress, DHEA decreases corticosteroid levels, thus effectively functioning as an immune system stimulator and a stress buffer.

But stress management—vitally important though it is—appears to merely scratch the surface of DHEA's capacity to re-arm us immunologically.

Raymond Daynes, Ph.D., emminent DHEA researcher from the University of Arizona, has done a neat trick in the vaccination of mice. A crisply functioning immune system needs to be competent at making freshly designed antibodies to fight new diseases it has never met before. But old rodents aren't very good at this. (And neither are old people.) A seventy-five-year-old man or woman's immune system will still do a pretty good job at creating antibodies to combat an infection the body has been exposed to before. *New* diseases are quite another matter. Which is why vaccinations are markedly less effective for senior citizens than for young folks.

When Daynes took old mice and vaccinated them against diseases they had never had before, their immune systems proved almost totally ineffectual at creating the new antibodies required. He then gave the mice the virus the vaccine was designed against, and most of the unfortunate rodents died. So Daynes took another batch of old mice and carried out the same procedures but with the addition of DHEA. The mice suddenly became almost as proficient at forming new antibodies as young mice, and almost all of them lived.[5]

For ethical reasons, one obviously can't give old people viruses, but two university studies have been under way to determine whether supplementation with DHEA will have the same effect on human ability to form novel antibodies as it does in mice. The results have not yet been published, but scientists involved in this research say that they appear overwhelmingly positive.

To return to animals, old mice that suffer burn injuries typically die. Supplementation with DHEA greatly increases the survival rate. When rats were inoculated with a virulent West Nile virus and then subjected to the stress of immersion in cold water, two thirds of them died. Treatment with DHEA significantly reduced the mortality rate.[6] It is now thought that DHEA stimulates the body's production of T-cells, B-cell lymphocytes, and macrophages. Our thymus gland, which is responsible for the production of T-cells, begins to shrink after we reach adulthood. One study now indicates that DHEA slows the rate of shrinkage. If more confirming evidence for that is found, then DHEA will fall into place alongside HGH and melatonin as a vital trio geared toward protecting the single most important organ of the immune system.

What Is DHEA?

A bit above waist level, a pair of small, yellowish organs rest on top of your kidneys. They're called the adrenal glands. The center of the glands produces adrenalin, your fight-or-flight hormone. The outer layer or cortex of the adrenals has as its prime production DHEA, a steroid out of which the adrenals manufacture a wide spectrum of other steroid hormones, including aldosterone, which preserves minerals in the body, and cortisone, which controls immune responses and affects energy and mineral metabolism. The adrenal glands also make both male and female sex hormones from DHEA but in much lower amounts than the reproductive organs do.

DHEA itself is made by the adrenals from cholesterol, an enormously useful substance, which has become a byword for cardiovascular danger to Americans (to an extent not readily supported by the facts). There is never any shortage of cholesterol even in old age, so DHEA's faltering production as the years pass is obviously the result of some difficulty in its manufacture rather than a shortage of raw material.

I should point out that, although, for the sake of simplicity, I refer to DHEA throughout the book, the hormone is actually most readily measured as DHEA sulfate (DHEAS). DHEA levels can shift wildly from hour to hour. DHEAS, a more stable form of DHEA, which has storage depots in the bone marrow and the adrenals, fluctuates far less widely. Consequently, when lab tests are done, it corresponds very nicely—even at its lower levels in the blood—with the total quantity of all forms of DHEA in the body. As for supplementation, both forms of the hormone are used, and there remains a controversy over which is more appropriate. Both appear to be effective, but since DHEA has been more widely used and is proven effective, I would recommend it.

And, indeed, whatever the diverse mechanisms by which the pro-longevity hormones extend active immunological life, there seems to be no doubt now of their fundamental efficacy. Old animals regain the normal vitality exhibited by much younger animals when their supplies of HGH, DHEA, and (as you'll see in the next chapter) melatonin are replaced. The considerable amount of research already done in people strongly supports the idea that we respond just as the animals do.

Cancer

If heart disease is catastrophic, cancer is fearful. Here, once again, the evidence is mainly in animals, but impressive nonetheless.

DHEA has caused cancer to regress in studies on dogs and cats. In mice, it has inhibited both spontaneous breast cancer and chemically induced tumors of the lung and colon.

In humans, small studies have shown gastric cancer, prostate cancer, and bladder cancer to be associated with low levels of DHEA. A much larger study conducted for nine years in the 1960s on the Isle of Guernsey and reported in *Lancet* in 1971 found only slightly lower DHEA levels in women who subsequently contracted breast cancer but significantly lower levels of androsterone, a steroid hormone made from DHEA.[7] The jury is still out on whether DHEA supplementation will help prevent breast cancer, but it certainly does no harm.

MEMORY AND INTELLECTUAL ABILITY

Poorer memory in old age is one of the similarities of mice and men. Therefore, it's encouraging to report that old mice given DHEA in the course of training improved their ability to remember until they were almost as efficient at it as young mice.

Memory difficulty is an aspect of aging that has been extremely hard to change positively.

Another indication that poor intellectual function among some older folks may be related to falling DHEA levels comes from a study by Daniel Rudman, M.D., showing that men in nursing homes had far lower blood levels of DHEAS than men of the same age who were living independantly. Forty percent of the nursing home residents versus only 6 percent of the men who lived in their own homes had subnormal levels for their age. Men who were senile or who were totally unable to care for themselves were even more likely to have low DHEAS. Levels were subnormal in 80 percent of the latter.[8]

Many scientists now believe that DHEA, which is six and a half times more abundant in normal brain tissue than in other bodily tissue, will prove to be important in the preservation of a vigorously functioning brain. Dr. Eugene Roberts added low concentrations of DHEA to nerve cell tissue cultures and found he could "increase the number of neurons, their ability to establish contacts between neurons, and their differentiation into highly functional brain cells."

HOW MUCH DHEA DOES ONE NEED?

DHEA conforms perfectly to the principal that this book adheres to. When it comes to anti-aging medicine, more isn't automatically better: The right amount is that which the body was made to handle. In practice, that often means that each individual should take a supplemental dose sufficient to bring his or her levels up to where they were when he or she was young. This is certainly the best procedure for prescribing DHEA, and, happily, we know roughly what normal levels are at different ages. (See Table 6.1.)

How much below the normal level for a twenty-year-old you may be depends on your age and also upon your individuality. Remember that, if used properly, DHEA is a very safe substance. However, it was, until recently, a prescription item. I think it's best if you still treat it as such and, therefore, establish a bona fide doctor/patient relationship with a physician who appreciates the value of hormone replacement. He or she will be able to have your levels tested, as I describe below.

In the last year, the Food and Drug Administration has decided to step back from regulating DHEA, and the Drug Enforcement Administration, which for a while was defining it as an anabolic steroid and, therefore, a controlled substance, has also backed off. You can now get DHEA without a prescription at most health-food stores and many drug stores. I can not guarantee the quality of all the products now marketed as DHEA. One company whose DHEA

Table 6.1
Standard Levels of DHEA in Men and Women

MEN		WOMEN	
Age	DHEAS Range (ng/ml)	Age	DHEAS Range (ng/ml)
15–39	1500–5500	15–29	1000–5000
40–49	1000–4000	30–39	600–3500
50–59	600–3000	40–49	400–2500
>60	300–2000	>50	200–1500

(Source: Orentreich, N. et al. "Age Changes and Sex Differences in Serum Dehydroepiandrosterone Sulfate Concentrations throughout Adulthood," *Journal of Clinical Endocrinology and Metabolism*, 59[3]1984, 551–555.)

is of standard potency and purity is Life Enhancement Products, Inc., in Petaluma, California. They sell powder-containing capsules. I believe more effective absorption can be obtained with the micronized form of DHEA—tiny granules suspended in oil-filled capsules. The main manufacturer of DHEA in the United States is Diosynth in Chicago, which is owned by Axzo, a large manufacturer of nutrients in the Netherlands. Their reputation stands very high, and I suspect that most of the companies that are currently distributing DHEA in this country are purchasing the hormone from Diosynth.

When taken by mouth, DHEA is rapidly absorbed into the bloodstream. The large increase that results is followed, within an hour or so, by a rapid drop to an intermediate level as DHEA is stored as DHEAS. Those storage depots are then drawn on as the body needs more or less DHEA throughout the day.

Before your doctor prescribes DHEA for you, he or she will certainly want to have a clinical laboratory measure your blood levels of DHEAS. I believe that, after you have been supplementing for a month or two, you should have your blood levels checked again.

Interpretation of laboratory reports of DHEAS blood levels is complicated by the fact that different laboratories report their results in different types of measurement units. Here's how to make these differences understandable.

Results are sometimes reported in nanograms per milliliter (ng/ml), in which case the results will usually range from 3,000 to 5,000 in vigorous young adults and can be as low as 200 to 500 in elderly or highly stressed people.

Other laboratories report their results as micrograms per milliliter (mcg/ml), which simply means that the decimal point has been moved three numbers to the left. Instead of 3,000 to 5,000 ng/ml, the same level of DHEAS is reported as 3 to 5 mcg/ml. Low levels will go down to 0.2 mcg/ml.

A third method of reporting is in micrograms per deciliter (mcg/dl). A deciliter is 100 milliliters, so the decimal point goes back two places to the right, and desirable ranges vary from 300 to 500, with deficient levels down to 20 or 30. By looking for these units of measurement on the report form, you can make a proper interpretation of the results, although it is usually quite obvious from the number of zeros.

I have found that a desirable range for a twenty-five-year-old is approximately 3,000 to 5,000 ng/ml for men and 2,500 to 3,000 for women. I aim for those levels by supplementing DHEA by mouth. The usual requirement is 25 to 50 milligrams (mg) of DHEA per day for women and 50 to 100 mg per day for men. Some practitioners prescribe up to 200 mg per day without any apparent problems, but I have seen such good results using the lower, more naturally occurring replacement doses that I see no reason to use more. Naturally the age and physical condition of an individual will affect the amount required to bring his or her level into the desirable range, but surprisingly often that amount will be within the range described above, whatever the initial levels of DHEAS were. You should measure and regulate your dose by having your blood levels checked before you begin replacement therapy and one month after you've started. After that—assuming you've now reached the desirable range—having your levels checked once a year should be sufficient.

In early research studies very high doses of DHEA, sometimes up to 3,000 mg per day, were given. Side effects were not common but did occur. Women must show more caution than men when taking such excessive doses because DHEA in excess has a testosterone-like effect. Normal replacement doses are often extremely helpful for women healthwise, but too much could theoretically cause the growth of facial hair, a cosmetic alteration that very few women, in my experience, regard as an improvement.

The key to safe and desirable results for DHEA, as for all the hormones described in this book, is rigid moderation. Go for the physiological dose. There is absolutely no evidence that a blood level that was good for you at twenty-five will harm you at age sixty-five and—as we've seen—a great deal of evidence that it will help you.

Don't be tempted by the notion of megadoses. With hormones, more is almost never better. This is a hormone, not a vitamin. You can take twenty times the normal intake of vitamin C daily and suffer no harm—indeed, you may do yourself a great deal of good. *This ambitious approach does not apply to hormones.*

A caution for men is also in order. Even a slight increase in testosterone is risky for men with prostate cancer, the likelihood of which is indicated by a significantly elevated prostate-specific antigen (PSA) test. Therefore, men with a definite or tentative diagnosis of prostate cancer should probably only begin DHEA supplementation under the guidance of a physician who is thoroughly familar with prostate problems and willing to follow up their condition with periodic examinations and lab tests.

For a much more extensive discussion of prostate problems and a cautious approach to them, see Chapter Ten, where I discuss the advantages and disadvantages of supplementing directly with the main male sex hormone, testosterone.

MAKING CHOICES IN A REAL WORLD

The final word on DHEA's safety, whether for men or women, remains very similar to that which we shall be saying for nearly all the hormones discussed in this book. There is no good evidence so far to suggest that hormones given in the amounts that the human body naturally secretes between the ages of twenty and thirty will prove harmful to the vast majority of individuals who take them. Nothing is perfectly safe. It is always conceivable that in a particular individual the metabolic balance is so delicately poised that even the addition of a substance entirely natural to the body in quantities that are also natural will, nonetheless, do him or her harm.

But just living is an act of balancing risks and advantages. As the hormone revolution that is now upon us unfolds, most of us as we get older will have to make a choice between accepting the small risk involved in hormonal supplementation for the sake of its substantial advantages and taking life as it comes to us—a course of action that has its own set of advantages and disadvantages. As far as dehydroepiandrosterone is concerned, all the evidence we now possess points toward a body of remarkable health improvements made possible by reversing nature's inclination to deprive you of it as you age.

The Myth of Precursors

If you want to obtain DHEA indirectly, you can go into the health-food marketplace and buy herbal products such as Mexican yam derivatives that contain alleged precursor molecules that could potentially be made into DHEA in your body. Unfortunately the ability of your body to make DHEA from precursor molecules is precisely what's diminishing with age. As you saw, cholesterol is the hormone's main precursor in your body, but that doesn't mean eating a lot of eggs will raise your DHEA level.

And, although some people do report an increased sense of well-being from taking herbal precursors to DHEA, that may result from other stimulant activity that some of these products have. The only proven method of raising your DHEA level is by taking DHEA itself. Any other approach is almost certainly a waste of time and money.

CHAPTER SEVEN

The Melatonin Magical Mystery Tour

MELATONIN, MELATONIN! EVERYONE'S BEEN TALKING ABOUT IT
for the past year. Millions of people have been taking it,
and health-food stores advertise it in their plate-glass win-
dows. Is it as important as Drs. Pierpaoli and Regelson
claimed in their bestselling book, *The Melatonin Miracle*?

My reply is a thunderous maybe. This is a very important hormone. The more we learn, the more impressive it
becomes. The six-million-dollar question is: Will supplementation with melatonin increase your life span by 25
percent? That's what it's done in mice. There are good reasons for thinking it might do something quite similar in
people. But for a definitive answer, you'll just have to wait
until 2050. The difficulty with doing longevity studies in
humans is that people live so darn long.

That said, I'm still going to devote the next two chapters to discussing this mighty maybe. Whether melatonin
does or doesn't add twenty years to your life, it's most
certainly going to improve it in ways that are well worth
having, and, in combination with the other pro-longevity
hormones, its value is unquestionable. As you'll see, its
usefulness as an enhancer of the immune system is very

significant. That's a property we're seeing in all of the pro-longevity hormones. The last twenty years of research has made it clear that relationships between the many endocrine glands and the immune system are unusually close. And let me put it quite bluntly—if I haven't done so already—when it comes to outfoxing death, a powerful, vigilant, ceaselessly active immune system is the master defender. Nothing except the beating of your heart is more critical to your continued survival.

In addition to its immunological effects, melatonin deserves serious attention for its impressive potency as an antioxidant. I'm sure that most of you will have seen that term used again and again in magazine articles and news reports. Vitamins C and E are antioxidants. Beta carotene and selenium are antioxidants. The B-complex vitamins enhance antioxidant protection, as do copper, zinc, manganese, and many other antioxidants. Fruits and vegetables are filled with antioxidants. What these antioxidants are supposed to be protecting you from are molecules called free radicals. Each of the antioxidants will offer a slightly different approach to free radical protection.

Until the last decade, this whole theory of free radical damage to the body and antioxidant protection was somewhat speculative. It has now entered the mainstream of medical knowledge, and it is widely conceded that free radicals play an extremely significant role in the aging process.

The antioxidant theory of aging was proposed four decades ago by Dr. Denham Harman. He had observed that radiation produced damage in the human body very similar to the effects of aging. What the radiation was doing was something that—thankfully at a slower rate—occurs in all our bodies as a normal consequence of simply living. You see, oxygen, which is the very basis of our form of life, without which we cannot live or produce energy, is also a bad guy.

In the normal process of cell metabolism, oxygen is used to burn or oxidize fuel from the food we eat in order to produce energy. As a by-product of this oxidative process, highly reactive and damaging forms of oxygen called free radicals are produced. When susceptible molecules in our cells encounter free radicals, they break apart and are otherwise damaged. If you ever took chemistry in high school, you'll remember that a molecule is composed of two or more atoms held together by electron bonds. The electrons are paired, with a balanced electrical charge that creates a stable molecular structure. In the course of reacting with oxygen, many molecules lose or gain an electron and become electrically unbalanced. This unbalanced molecule is called a free radical and its instantaneous desire is to combine with (oxidize) any other atom in its vicinity. It can do this in a nanosecond, a billionth of a second, and the result in your body is damage to tissues, to cells, and to the very RNA and DNA in the nucleus of your cells that forms the genetic core program of life. Trillions of these free radical reactions are occurring in our bodies daily and without the protection of antioxidants, molecules that combine with free radicals in order to neutralize them, we would be in very deep trouble. In fact, we would be in much the same situation as a person who is exposed to a killing blast of nuclear radiation, which overwhelms all antioxidant defenses and creates widespread molecular destruction in the body.

Well, much of aging is an accumulation of free radical damage. And research has indicated that a long list of diseases from cancer and heart disease to Alzheimer's, Parkinson's, and arthritis are caused in part or in whole by free radicals.

Thus the discovery of any important new antioxidant is of singular significance. Antioxidants make cells and molecules "bullet proof" against free radicals. Melatonin may be a particularly crucial addition to the antioxidant armory.

Apparently it is one of the few powerful antioxidants that can pass through the blood-brain barrier,[1] an anatomical feature designed to protect our brain from chemical or bacterial and toxic assault. Since our brain is much more subject to free radical molecular damage than any other part of our body, it could easily turn out that the significant portion of the aged population that shows a decline in brain function is experiencing the effects of declining levels of melatonin.

Various studies have shown that melatonin is one of—if not the most—vigorous antioxidant protector. But now, let's move from the molecular level to the larger picture; let's see just what a remarkable hormone melatonin is in the total scope of life.

MASTER OF THE STAGES OF LIFE

Melatonin is the major hormone produced by our pineal gland. The pineal is a tiny cone-shaped body buried deep within our brain. Cloaked in utter darkness, it is, nonetheless, designed to be sensitive to light. Indeed, the pineal is the master of our circadian rhythm, the whole process by which we are attuned to the cycles of day and night, light and dark. In animals the pineal, through its light sensitivity, controls the body's response to the seasons. Bears hibernate, birds migrate, animals of all sorts mate during a restricted time of year. The pineal gland is a miraculous master controller of those cycles.

The Hindus referred to the pineal as "the third eye" and portrayed it as one of the seven chakras or centers of vital energy, which are arranged along the central axis of the body. Located at the apex of the head, it was thought by them to be the supreme or crown chakra and a source of bodily harmony. Rene Descartes, the seventeenth-century French philosopher, said the pineal was the seat of the soul (and found himself in theological hot water). In modern western medicine, however, the pineal was for a long time much neglected. Nobody knew what it did, and, until 1958, when Dr. Aaron Lerner, a Yale dermatologist, published an article in the *Journal of the American Chemical Society*, few people were aware that the hormone he dubbed melatonin even existed.[2]

Now we know that our bodies would go haywire without melatonin, and the fact that the pineals of the very old produce it in much-reduced quantities is a contributor to many of the health hazards of age.

Is the pineal actually the clock that regulates aging? Does it determine the stages of life? This is a hypothesis that now has much to support it. Certainly melatonin production has an impact on every stage of our life. Newborns produce very little of it. Then, at about three months of age—which is the stage of development when they start sleeping longer stretches at night and being more alert during the day—melatonin levels rise. From about the age of one, melatonin levels are more or less constant for a decade. Then, just before puberty, they go down sharply. Recent studies have demonstrated that this decline is the body's signal to the sex glands to set sexual maturation in motion. So clear is the signal meant to be, that a child who maintains unusually high levels of melatonin will experience a delay in the onset of pubescence. There have actually been rare cases, in which the melatonin level is so uncharacteristically high in adolescence that sexual maturation simply does not occur!

From adolescence to early middle age, melatonin levels more or less plateau. But somewhere around forty-five years of age, melatonin begins a steep decline, thus joining the ranks of the other declining hormones—estrogen, testosterone, DHEA, and human growth hormone. The endocrine hormones are essential for vital, energetic lives, but our bodies phase them out as the years advance. By the time they're sixty, most people are producing less than half the melatonin they produced at twenty; by their late seventies, many people are producing hardly any melatonin at all. We know that the broken sleep patterns of many older men and women are a consequence of this deficit, but it also seems clear that the impairment of many of our most critical glands is also related to this shortage. The truth is that something vital is interrupted in people when the pineal gland's functioning declines. Our circadian rhythms (day/night cycles) are a crucial part of our nature and our relationship to the planet we live on and the sun we orbit. We are creatures of the light and the darkness, constructed for activity in daylight and rest at night.

Melatonin is necessary for a restful night's sleep. Securely protected in the center of our heads, the pineal gland nonetheless knows all about light. When light reaches the retina of our eyes, the eye communicates the degree of light or dark to the pineal by a complicated pathway through the nervous system. Light inhibits the production of melatonin. Therefore, the hormone is mostly produced at night, starting around 11:00 P.M. and peaking between 2:00 and 3:00 A.M. This nocturnal production promotes sleepiness. In the last few years, insomniacs have been alerted to the drug-free benefits of the hormone, and travelers have discovered with relief that a simple melatonin tablet can relieve jet lag.

If melatonin is so important to our daily physical harmony and so reliably marks out the different stages of life, it wouldn't be at all surprising to find that it has some role to play in the final stage, the stage of our decline. In fact, when we reach our mid-forties, the pineal begins to undergo rapid aging, and the instrument of its action, melatonin, is progressively secreted at markedly lower levels.

Is melatonin a pro-longevity hormone? Would we be better off if our levels remained closer to what we had in youth?

MOUSE AMAZEMENT

It's time to take a look at what happens to animals when their melatonin levels go up or down.

Much of what we know is due to the very inventive research of scientists at the Center for Experimental Pathology in Locarno, Switzerland. Walter Pierpaoli, M.D., coauthor of last year's best-selling melatonin book, was one of the leading experimenters. In 1985 he and his colleagues decided to test the effect of administering melatonin to old mice. The first experiment involved healthy male mice nineteen months old. Since this breed lives to twenty-four months, this was roughly the equivalent of dealing with sixty-five-year-old humans. The mice were divided into two groups, with the first group receiving melatonin-laced drinking water and the second group regular tap water.

Dr. Pierpaoli assumed there would be improvements in immune function in the melatonin group. Even in 1985, good evidence existed for melatonin's ability to enhance the immune system. What actually occurred, however, was simply astonishing. The untreated mice, of course, marched on into late old age. They lost muscle, developed bald patches in their fur, cataracts on their eyes, and all the other solemn indicators of their approaching end. They became increasingly inactive as their life force wound down.

Meanwhile, the mice on melatonin were not getting older but apparently younger. Their fur had become thick and shiny, their eyes were clear, their muscles firm, and in activity and energy they resembled far younger mice. Moreover, they went on living. The untreated mice began to die at around twenty-four months. The melatonin mice survived an extra six months, the equivalent in human terms of living past a hundred.[3]

According to Dr. Pierpaoli, the mice showed one other remarkable quality: Not only did the treated mice live longer, they remained healthy, disease-free, and relatively vigorous until virtually the end of their lives. Tests indicated that their immune function was similar to young mice, and their thyroid function, which generally shows signs of decline in older animals, also remained youthful. One last indicator spelled youthfulness. The melatonin mice remained sexually active until almost the end of their very long lives. Do centenarians pursue the opposite sex? They do if they're melatonin-treated mice.

For mice, here was the fountain of youth. Melatonin had shown itself capable of rejuvenating at least three systems: the endocrine, the immune, and the reproductive. Consequently it extended life. The theory that the pineal gland might in some way be a major regulator of the body's overall, age-related functioning had definitely received support. And, of course, such a wide range of benefits had done far more than increase longevity. These mice had lived again in the happy vigor of youth.

Dr. Pierpaoli's team decided to take their research one step further and actually transfer young pineal glands into old mice. Surgically it was too difficult to put these glands into the mice's brains as replacements for their old pineal glands, so they implanted them in the thymus, the immune-system gland lying behind the breastbone. Since the thymus is fed by the same nerves as the pineal, this seemed a logical location.[4]

The results were interesting. The old mice did live three months longer than their untreated brethren, but this was only half the increase in longevity brought about by the simple ingestion of melatonin. It occurred to Dr. Pierpaoli that this might be because the animals still retained their old pineals. If the pineal is the regulator, the controller of the aging clock, the conductor of the symphony of glands that permits life, then it seemed probable that two pineal glands, one old and one young would produce discordance in the music. The final demonstration of the pineal gland's potency was still ahead.

In the early 1990s, techniques of microsurgery finally made it possible to conduct pineal transplantations within the brain of the mouse. That's more difficult than one can easily imagine, since the pineal is extremely small—pea-sized in a human, microscopic in a mouse. Nonetheless, surgery was successfully done on groups of four-month-old and eighteen-month-old mice. Each old mouse was given the pineal of a young mouse, and each young mouse an old pineal.[5]

The results were as bizarre as anything dreamed up in Frankenstein's lab. After several months of adjustment, it became obvious that the "young" mice were rapidly aging, while the "old" mice had become young again. The two groups rapidly passed each other moving in opposite directions. The young mice, decrepit before their time, all died in middle age. The rejuvenated older mice lived to thirty-three months, the equivalent in human terms of 105 years. Although Pierpaoli and Regelson do not ask the question in their book, I cannot help wondering what would have happened if, some months before the little rodents' eventual demise, they had taken the old mice, removed their second pineal glands, and given them yet a third pineal gland—yet another young one. Would they have been rejuvenated a second time? Would they have begun again, fur glossy, sex drive restored, and added yet another six or seven months to their record-breaking lifespan? How many times could such a step be taken? What are the limits of longevity, if the pineal should prove to be its crucial element?

Can we extrapolate these fairly earth-shattering achievements in mouse medicine to human beings? Should we order the champagne and send out the invitations for our hundredth-birthday parties now? Although I'm firmly convinced that most of the readers of this book have an extremely good likelihood of reaching a hundred or more, I wouldn't plan the celebration simply on the basis of melatonin. As I'll be showing you in the pages to come, this is a powerful hormone. But no one knows if it will do for human longevity what it has done for our little rodent friends. People are a great deal more complex than mice, they live a great deal longer, and the pattern of their aging is necessarily different from that of a mouse. If it turns out that folks who take supplemental melatonin from middle age on increase their life span by 25 percent, then no one will be celebrating more vigorously than the authors of this book. I think we should hold that speculation in reserve.

Let's look instead at the unquestioned benefits of melatonin.

SMART IMMUNITY

Whether or not the pineal gland turns out to be the body's aging clock, there is very little doubt that its hormone, melatonin, does a magnificent job of priming your immune system.

The immune system is one of the most "intelligent" enterprises in the human body. Specifically, it knows who we are and what is and what isn't us. That's much more difficult than you might, at first blush, think it to be. The living cells of your body have tremendous similarities to all the other living organisms in the world around us. We live in symbiosis with an enormous number of bacteria. They enter our mouths and our noses, they prosper on the surface of our skin, they inhabit the interior world of our intestines. Some of them are beneficial, some alien but relatively benign, and many of them harmful or disastrously malignant. Before the age of antibiotics, infections were one of the leading causes of death. But antibiotics are simply an extra defense that we employ when our natural defenses are on the verge of being overwhelmed. Our first line of defense is our immune system, which we already have within us.

At any time in human history, death would have come upon us rather quickly if it were not for the incomparable sophistication with which our immune system defends us. Confronted daily with thousands of different bacterial intruders, it knows what's us and what isn't us—what to attack and what to leave alone. Our immune system can't attack everything that's not us, of course. If it did, how would we eat food?

Thus, our immune system is a system of identification possessing the power of discrimination and judgment, as well as providing a murderously effective team of killer cells. It is the intelligence corps that identifies the enemy, the general who decides whether to attack, and the army that takes out the tough guys as needed. Of the hormones discussed in this book, three—DHEA, human growth hormone, and melatonin—have demonstrated a capacity to radically upgrade our immune system as it ages. Just as these three hormones seem to give us the strength and energy we had when young, so they give back to our immune system the organizing intelligence and aggressive vigor that was natural to it in our youth.

How big is the immune difference between young and old? Well, the odds of a teenager dying of cancer is about 1 in 25,000. The likelihood that an infectious disease other than AIDS will bring his young life to a close is about 1 in 2,000,000. Once you're over seventy, however, you have about a 1-in-8 chance of dying of cancer and a 1-in-30 chance of dying of an infectious disease.

If you're planning to live in good health and for a long time, the place to start is your immune system.

Melatonin has earned its spurs in a host of medical studies conducted since the mid-1980s. We shouldn't be surprised, for it is the only substance apart from human growth hormone (and possibly DHEA) that has shown evidence of being able to regenerate the thymus gland, the original seat of immune system function. You'll remember that in Chapter Four, when we were discussing HGH and immunity, we spoke about the thymus's virtual disappearance with age and the highly damaging effect that has on immunity. Back in the 1970s, the pineal research team in Locarno, Switzerland, demonstrated that the thymus glands of even young animals would begin to shrivel up if the pineal gland was removed. That was pretty telling evidence of a connection that nobody had suspected until then. And that connection has held up, for in the experiment we just discussed in which young pineals were put into old mice and old pineals into young ones, the thymus glands of the young mice soon began to wither and the thymus glands of the old mice grew and regenerated.

The experiment in which old mice had melatonin added to their drinking water also offered telling evidence. The thymus glands of those mice increased in size and began more actively producing T-cell lymphocytes, called the killer cells of the immune system—they kill ineffective microorganisms and destroy cancer cells. Let's quickly look at three other examples of enhanced immune function brought about by melatonin.

Melatonin: Enhancing Survival

Interestingly enough, a double-blind study[6] conducted by Virginia Utermohlen at Cornell University demonstrated that melatonin is even capable of enhancing the immune response of young adults. Ten male college students were given either 20 mg of melatonin or a placebo for a week. When the study was being conducted a virus was going around the campus, and many of the men participating had a cold. Those receiving melatonin produced 250 percent more salivary IgA, an immune antibody protein that helps protect against colds and upper respiratory infections.

Two mouse studies showed vastly increased resistance to severe infection after melatonin was administered. In one,[7] the mice were given a sublethal dose of encephalomyocarditis virus. This was usually not enough to kill mice, but the researchers went further and stressed the mice by confining them for several hours a day in tubes perforated with air holes. Immune function declined correspondingly. Half the mice were then given melatonin, and the researchers sat back to see what happened. The untreated mice fared very badly—in the end, only 6 percent of them survived. But by the end of the study, 82 percent of the melatonin-treated mice had overcome the combination of physical and mental stress they had been exposed to and were still alive.

In the other mouse study,[8] a mixed group of young and old mice were injected with encephalitis—a virus that causes an often fatal brain infection—again accompanied by stress confinement. Half of each age group were then given melatonin. Of the untreated mice, only 6 percent of the young and none of the old survived. Of the treated mice, 39 percent of the young and 56 percent of the old survived, an interesting and rare advantage for the old that has not yet been explained.

The Army of Immunity

These various research demonstrations are all well and good, but *how* does melatonin support immune function? The most promising finding was made in 1995, when scientists discovered that melatonin links up with a type of immune cell known as the T-helper cell, which aids in the action of antibodies.[9] In fact, it turns out that there are melatonin receptor sites on the surfaces of those cells. Our body is so precisely designed that all cells have receptors that are specifically crafted to receive the molecules that are going to visit them.

Imagine a space ship fitting precisely into the mother ship's landing dock. If T-helper cells have landing docks for melatonin, that means melatonin was always intended to go there and presumably was always intended to influence the immune system—a highly significant finding. And, if both melatonin production and T-helper cells decline with age—and they do—then, considering melatonin's demonstrated effects on immune function, it's pretty certain this isn't coincidental.

The T-helper cells are one particular form of the T-cells that are most important to our immune system. These T-cells actually originate in our bone marrow, but then they migrate to our thymus gland for their higher education. One T-cell will learn that it must respond to the herpes virus, another recognizes and attacks tuberculosis, a third goes after one particular upper respiratory infection. Every T-cell is trained to be a specialist, and, after graduation, they go forth prepared to fight and die for you. There are billions of T-cells in your body right now, on the lookout for their designated enemies.

Your body has two main varieties: T-killer cells and T-helper cells. The T-helper cells are the commanding officers in this army. Once a bacterial or viral enemy is spotted, the T-helper cells signal for the troops. Chemical messages transmitted by substances called cytokines tell the body which T-cells are needed, and, in a matter of hours or days, millions of exact copies of the specialized T-killer cells that target that particular invader are produced and directed to the site of infection, where they go into battle. Since most of us live fairly long lives, you can be confident that your T-cell army has won thousands of victories.

If melatonin supports the T-helper cells, then we have at least a partial explanation for its unquestionable capacity to enhance our immune system. Since it also appears to regenerate the thymus, our immune system's original powerhouse, it may work synergistically with human growth hormone to keep us disease free as we age. Certainly these are convincing scientific explanations for the tremendous increases in immunity that both hormones have separately produced. When we talk about devising a comprehensive plan of hormonal supplementation in Chapter Fifteen, we'll ask ourselves what is the likely result of combining so many powerful substances.

THE CANCER CONNECTION

As I pointed out earlier, modern medical science has arrived rather firmly at the conclusion that cancer is in large part a disease caused by failure of the immune system. This is, of course, the reason why it is, by and large, a disease of aging. Breast cancer has become fearfully common in our society, and many people have read magazine articles and listened to media discussions of the principal risk factors. Having no children, having the first child late in life, not breast-feeding, having relatives with breast cancer, early menstruation, late menopause—the list is long. But the factor that correlates most strongly with a woman's likelihood of contracting the disease is her age. And this simple, unavoidable risk is actually at the very top of the list for most other cancers as well.

Thus it seems probable that the best way (other than dying young) not to get cancer is to keep your immune system as much like that of a young person as you possibly can. I believe that following the suggestions in this book will allow most of us to do just that—if not forever, then at least until we reach our nineties. Remember that in the *normal* process of aging, unsupplemented by hormones, the immune system declines dramatically in our seventies.

Melatonin is bound to be important in this struggle. If, indeed, the pineal gland proves to be our aging clock, then it may be the most important of all. For the moment, however, let's look at some of the very suggestive research that has been carried out on the relationship between melatonin and cancer.

First, I'd like to recall the experiences of one isolated physician, Dr. Kenneth Starr. In 1963, just five years after melatonin had been identified, Dr. Starr gave large intravenous doses of it to a young man with a tumor in his leg that had spread to his lymph nodes. The treatment resulted in a complete remission. Starr had successes with a number of other cancer patients, but being an "unimportant" private physician without access to the major medical journals, his work was soon forgotten.

He was actually not the first pioneer. As far back as the early 1900s, there have been doctors who thought that some unknown substance in the pineal gland blocked cancer growth. A number of these physicians gave ground-up pineal glands to cancer patients and reported positive responses.

There was no real follow-up to these early successes. It is easy to blame the cancer researchers, but it probably wouldn't be fair. They have pursued cancer cures up and down thousands of blind alleys, and science is complicated. Now, however, melatonin's time has arrived.

In 1980 an American scientist named Lawrence Tamarkin injected rats with DMBA, a potent carcinogen that stimulates the growth of breast tumors. He then administered a daily dose of melatonin to some of the rodents. After ninety days, 50 percent of the untreated rats had breast tumors. Not one of the melatonin-treated animals had developed a tumor. Tamarkin then stopped giving melatonin, and eventually 20 percent of the melatonin group developed tumors as well.[10]

Naturally one wonders if results like this could occur in the human female.

Breast Cancer and Melatonin

One of the leading investigators in this field is David Blask, M.D., Ph.D., working out of the Mary Imogene Bassett Research Institute in Cooperstown, New York. In 1986 Blask attempted to inhibit the growth of a virulent strain of breast cancer cells called MCF-7 cells. Cell lines like this are grown in a tissue culture from the actual tumor cells removed from a breast-cancer patient.

Blask and his team set up two groups of the MCF-7 cells, one receiving melatonin, the other not. The dosage of melatonin used was extremely large, a hundred times that found in the human bloodstream. To their disappointment, the growth of the cancer cells was not inhibited in the slightest. No matter how often they repeated the experiment, the result was the same.

At this stage, Blask might have abandoned the attempt, but it suddenly occurred to him to try a lesser dose. The normal practice in oncology research is to look for a maximum impact on cancer cells by giving a maximum dose. There is some logic to this when chemotherapy is being used, since chemotherapeutic agents are essentially chemical poisons not naturally present in the human body. Melatonin, however, is always naturally present, and when Blask began to dose his MCF-7 cells with melatonin at levels approximating the concentration normally present in the young human body, the results were dramatic. The growth of the breast cancer cells was blocked by 75 percent.[11]

Continued experimentation showed that the window of effectiveness was quite narrow. Concentrations of melatonin that were too much below or too far above the amount normally present in a healthy human body were equally ineffective.

Significant in itself, this research becomes still more telling if one remembers a study conducted at the National Institutes of Health (NIH) in 1978.[12] NIH scientists discovered that there was a direct statistical correlation between the incidence of breast cancer and the rate of pineal calcification as detected by X-rays of the skull. As the pineal gland ages, it frequently develops calcium deposits, a problem found in many organs of the body. This calcification stiffens a gland or organ and interferes with its activity.

Not everyone's pineal calcifies, however, and there are national differences. Countries—such as the United States—with a high rate of pineal calcification have high breast cancer rates. Countries with low rates of pineal calcification—Japan is an example—have low levels of breast cancer. As you might expect, pineal calcification is associated with low levels of melatonin. If, as Blask's research indicates, melatonin has a direct inhibitory effect on breast cancer cells, the circle is complete.

Can We Treat Breast Cancer with Melatonin?

I think it's very possible that melatonin supplementation will help in the prevention of breast cancer. But, for the hundreds of thousands of women who already have it, this approach may be too late.

In 1992, continuing with his work on breast cancer cells, David Blask decided to add melatonin to the already well established anti-breast-cancer drug, tamoxifen. Tamoxifen binds with estrogen receptors and inhibits their effects on cell growth. Since more than 60 percent of breast tumors are estrogen-sensitive, many women improve on tamoxifen. However, the drug is by no means side-effect free, and, in most cases, the initial positive effects begin to diminish with time. Blask hoped that adding melatonin would enable a lower dose of tamoxifen to be given while simultaneously enhancing the drug's effectiveness. This approach succeeded beyond his wildest dreams; when melatonin was used, the potency of tamoxifen was increased one hundred times.[13]

Paolo Lissoni, a neuroimmunologist from San Gerardo Hospital in Monza, Italy, was sufficently impressed with Blask's work to try the technique on fourteen women with advanced metastatic breast cancer who were not responding to treatment. All the women had been treated with tamoxifen before the study began and had either not responded or, after initial good effects, had begun to show diminished responses.

The women were receiving 20 mg of tamoxifen in the daytime and another 20 mg at night. In a 1995 article in the *British Journal of Cancer*, Lissoni reported an impressive series of results.[14] Four of the women had a 50 percent or greater reduction in the size of their tumors. Eight other women had no further increase in tumor size. And only two failed to respond to treatment.

Blask has been unable to get approval in the United States to try his therapy on humans, but, in a recent animal study, has been able to show significant improvement in mice given tamoxifen and melatonin in combination.

And in Prostate Cancer?

The male half of the population may enjoy equal cancer-fighting benefits from melatonin. In 1993 Dr. Christian Bartsch of the University of Tubingen in Germany reported that men with prostate cancer shared many accompanying hormonal abnormalities: low thyroid levels, low prolactin levels (prolactin stimulates the immune system), and high FSH levels (thereby promoting testicular activity). But what they most conspicuously showed was an utterly strange pattern of melatonin production. Instead of peaking at 2 or 3 A.M., their melatonin levels increased and decreased at unusual times, both in the afternoon and at night. Something was out of order in their pineal glands.

Prostate cancer is the most common form of cancer in men and second only to lung cancer in mortality. This year, 40,000 men, give or take a few, will die of it. Dr. David Blask has now followed up his breast cancer research by incubating human prostate cancer cells in melatonin. This resulted in a 50 percent inhibition of growth. Blask intends to proceed with further research in animals.

He is not alone. A study carried out by researchers at the University of Texas Medical School found that melatonin reduced the growth rate of prostatic tumors in rats by 50 percent. Such a result in men would certainly represent a sizable prolongation of life.

It remains to be seen whether melatonin's suspected influence over other hormonal systems is part of the reason for its benefits in both prostate and breast cancer. Both cancers, after all, are subject to hormonal stimulation. Estrogen and prolactin stimulate breast cancer, and testosterone stimulates prostate cancer. Both cancers can be arrested in their early stages but are much more dangerous once they've metastasized. And people who have either of these cancers tend to have unusually low levels of melatonin. But at this stage, we are merely speculating. It may turn out that all cancers are sensitive to melatonin therapy.

Dr. Lissoni Again

To date, the final piece of the melatonin/cancer puzzle is offered by that indefatigable Italian researcher, Dr. Paolo Lissoni. He has been tireless in pursuing the melatonin connection. In 1990, reasoning that the body calls on all parts of the immune system, not simply melatonin, to fight cancer, he decided to combine melatonin with interleukin-2. IL-2 is a natural part of our immune system, a signaling molecule that fosters immune cell growth. For many years, it has been one of the most investigated immunological approaches to fighting cancer, but there is a severe drawback. Given in doses high enough to inhibit a cancer, it is extremely toxic, and patients frequently die from side effects.

Lissoni wondered whether melatonin would reduce the toxicity effect. This proved to be the case. Equally significant, melatonin combined with IL-2 proved to be a great deal more effective than IL-2 alone. Lissoni and his team took eighty late stage cancer patients, put half on IL-2 and half on IL-2 plus melatonin. One year after the start of treatment, 46 percent of the patients in the IL-2 plus melatonin group were still alive versus only 15 percent of the patients in the IL-2 alone group.[15]

In 1994 Lissoni decided to try the melatonin/IL-2 therapy against one of the deadliest of all malignancies— late stage lung cancer. He ran his new combination therapy in a head-to-head competition with the combination of cis-platin and etoposide, a standard chemotherapeutic treatment for advanced lung cancer. At the end of the first year, 45 percent of those receiving melatonin/IL-2 were still alive, compared with only 19 percent of those on chemotherapy. The melatonin group also experienced fewer side effects.[16]

I think there's little doubt that melatonin is going to be vigorously researched as an anti-cancer agent in the future. This book, of course, is only peripherally concerned with cancer therapies. What impresses me about melatonin is the evidence that far from being just an effective natural sleeping potion, it is, as well, an essential part of the harmony of the human body. Like human growth hormone and DHEA, it resurrects something we cannot live for very long without: a vigorous and actively functioning immune system. As I said in an earlier chapter, Acquired Immune Deficiency Syndrome (AIDS) is a quick, sudden, and nasty demonstration of what overtakes us all eventually—the condition of immunological breakdown that, when it occurs in the old, could very appropriately be referred to as Natural Immune Deficiency Syndrome (NIDS).

NIDS isn't in the medical textbooks yet, but if the pro-longevity hormones continue to demonstrate such a gratifying abililty to halt it, we may someday find ourselves referring to NIDS as a disease that, once upon a time, older men and women inevitably succumbed to but which now they no longer need fear. Aging is a disease all right. Until very recently, medicine couldn't do a thing to treat it.

Evidently we're about to enter a different world.

CHAPTER EIGHT

Melatonin: Sleep King

MELATONIN'S CAPACITY TO AID IN SLEEP ENHANCEMENT IS NOT disputed by even the most skeptical critics of this hormone's new-found celebrity.

Since life without a good night's sleep is deprived living, this is one quality of the pineal's hormone well worth celebrating. How we sleep is controlled by our circadian cycle, the day-night cycle that synchronizes our hormone production, hunger, moods, body temperature, energy level, and, of course, sleep/wake patterns. This cycle runs twenty-four hours in length, roughly similar to our twenty-four-hour day, and it can change with age.

In fact, disturbances of the circadian cycle that affect the ability to get a good night's sleep are very common among older people. Not only do the elderly produce relatively low amounts of melatonin—the sleep messenger— they very commonly produce it out of phase. The most frequent old-age sleep disorder results when an individual starts producing melatonin too early in the evening and then stops producing it too early in the morning. Older folks with this problem have a tendency to fall asleep soon after dinner and then wake early, sometimes in the middle of the night, well before sunrise. Moreover, the quality of the sleep they get is often poor.

Consider, for a moment, what a good night's sleep is designed to do for you.

THE STAGES OF SLEEP

Sleep researchers, who have been vigorously delving into the mysteries of the kingdom of Nod, divide sleep into five separate stages: stages I, II, III, and IV, and REM sleep (rapid-eye-movement sleep)—the stage when you dream. As you dream, your eyes dart rapidly back and forth, as if you were following the action of your own private, interior movies—thus the name.

Stage I is the shallow sleep with which you begin a sleep cycle. Stage II is a little deeper, and is followed by Stages III and IV, which are really deep, non-dreaming (NREM) sleep. This deep sleep is generally regarded as the most restful sleep and probably does most to rejuvenate our energies for the coming day. In these stages, breathing is regular and slow, blood pressure goes down, and muscular movement is quite minimal. This is called delta sleep—even our brains slow down and brain waves, if recorded on EEG machines, show large, slow, smooth waves.

Because this deep sleep is so necessary to the replenishment and healing of our body, our sleep cycles pack as much of it in as possible during the early stages of rest, just in case our night's sleep is destined to be a short one. The cycles of sleep consist of sixty to one hundred minutes of NREM sleep followed by a significantly shorter period of dream sleep. As the night progresses, the NREM segments become somewhat shorter and the REM sleep longer. There are usually five to six cycles a night.

Older people seem to have a harder time staying in the deepest levels of NREM sleep. Since the body is believed to be carrying out a good deal of quiet repair and regeneration during those stages, this is unfortunate. Equally crippling, however, would be disruption of the REM dream stage. Without it, our mental functions deteriorate radically. Memory falters, learning becomes almost impossible, and psychological disorders occur. Sleep researchers believe that dreaming allows us to assimilate and cope with the various experiences we have had during our waking hours. Apparently our dreams allow us to clean up superfluous data and file away important information.

Without sufficient sleep, therefore, we are both physically exhausted and mentally somewhat disfunctional. Tens of millions of people attempt to address these problems by taking sleeping pills, and more than a third of the folks taking those prescription drugs are over sixty-five. Unfortunately, all the effective sleep-inducing drugs so far discovered disrupt normal sleep cycles and eventually make the problem worse. Benzodiazepines (which include Dalmane, Halcion, Valium, and Xanax) are among the worst offenders. Studies have shown that several months of benzodiazepine use can virtually abolish Stage III and IV sleep.[1]

If you have a sleep problem, what you need is a solution that reinforces rather than disrupts the normal patterns of sleep—and melatonin does just that.

What Melatonin Does

Richard Wurtman, M.D., a researcher at MIT, conducted a series of studies over ten years that demonstrated quite conclusively that even fractions of a milligram of melatonin can enhance sleep. His first studies used 240 milligrams—a huge dose by today's standards—and his subjects did, indeed, sleep—like rocks—and usually woke up feeling pretty groggy. Eventually Wurtman determined that as little as 0.3 milligrams would significantly decrease the amount of time a volunteer needed to fall asleep.[2]

The effective dose seems to vary widely from person to person, however. In my practice, an occasional elderly patient has taken 30 to 60 mg every night with good results and no side effects. Others have found that one mg or less is adequate and that more causes drowsiness the next day.

When you take a melatonin tablet, your pulse rate declines, your body temperature drops, and you begin to feel tranquil and drowsy. The gates of sleep begin to open. A recent study conducted at the Technion Medical School in Haifa, Israel, showed that men and women between the ages of sixty-eight and eighty who took melatonin cut the time they required to fall asleep by more than half (from forty minutes to fifteen), as well as reporting a more refreshing sleep.

If you have a problem sleeping, I recommend that you take between 1 and 5 mg of melatonin at your desired sleep time. Try the smaller dose first: it may be enough. Your goal is to get a solid night's sleep and wake up refreshed.

MELATONIN FOR LIFE?

Melatonin declines and so do we. Direct connection? Nobody knows for sure, but the evidence assembled so far— even though it's mostly the product of animal studies—is certainly interesting.

At the moment, my recommendation for people over forty-five is that they modestly supplement their bodies with melatonin. There is certainly no evidence of any kind to show that it can harm you. Thousands of people have taken it in clinical trials. Even when doses as high as several thousand milligrams were given daily for a month, there was no apparent toxicity. And that dose is thousands of times greater than what you'd take to maintain a youthful level of melatonin.

It would be better, of course, if there had been large-scale double-blind studies conducted over years that would have the capacity to accurately identify both benefits and negative effects. Having said that, we come back to the basic thesis of this book: What may or may not happen if you take megadoses of a hormone is inherently unpredictable, but what will happen if you take doses that approximate your own body's natural youthful levels is probably quite predictable. After all, this is what your body has been used to for decades.

Therefore, with melatonin as with other hormones, I recommend for my patients amounts that best approximate nature's original plan. When you are in your twenties, your melatonin blood level is at its adult peak of approximately 125 picograms. The level falls off very gradually, and, then in the mid-forties, a more dramatic decline begins. By the time you're eighty, you should be at approximately half your youthful peak.

The amount you should take will, therefore, vary quite naturally according to your age. My recommendation is that from age forty-five to fifty-four take from 0.2 to 1 mg. From fifty-five to sixty-four take 1 to 2 mg. From sixty-five to seventy-four take 2 to 3 mg; and from seventy-five on take 3 to 5 mg. But if you find a slightly larger dose produces more benefit, there is no evidence that it will harm you.

LONGEVITY OR JUST BETTER HEALTH?

We've already described a fairly comprehensive listing of major health benefits produced by melatonin. What I'm sure you'd like to know as much as I would is whether melatonin will radically restructure the body's aging clock and perhaps make it possible for us to live a healthy twenty to thirty years longer than the usual maximum of eighty to ninety years. I suppose the proper answer is that you and I and all the millions of other people who are taking melatonin now are guinea pigs in a great longevity experiment.

Doctors Regelson and Pierpaoli in their best-selling book, *The Melatonin Miracle*, have suggested that melatonin does reset the clock. In fact, the essence of their theory is that by taking a replacement dose of melatonin we essentially fool our bodies into thinking we're younger than we are. They have speculated that the pineal gland is the timer for aging.

The pineal gland begins to break down in our middle years. It shrinks, it loses many of its pinealocytes, the cells that produce melatonin and other compounds, and the system that transmits light signals from the retinas of the eyes to the pineal also begins to show wear and tear. As less melatonin and other pineal hormones are produced, it could well be that the body starts losing its ability to adjust to its environment. The loss of proper circadian rhythm appears to be related to the loss of many different kinds of essental metabolic adjustments. (For instance, older people have more difficulty adapting to extremes of heat and cold.)

Regelson and Pierpaoli's theory is that the slowing of melatonin production is a major signal to all the other hormone systems to begin slowing down. In effect, diminished melatonin is a message to self-destruct. The other glands, obedient to the pineal clock, then secrete less of their own critical hormones, and the process that we call aging proceeds on its less than merry way. Regelson and Pierpaoli cite the astonishing mouse studies that we described in the last chapter as evidence for this thesis.

Those studies are, of course, also evidence for the far more pleasing idea that supplemental melatonin can cause the pineal gland to age more slowly and that most of the other crucial hormonal systems will follow suit, thus effectively slowing aging throughout the body. Such a theory is potent but unproven stuff. But there's no harm that I can see in whistling optimistically as we take our melatonin tablets. This hormone is a mighty antioxidant, a vigorous enhancer of our immune system, and an extraordinary cancer fighter, and virtually guarantees a good night's sleep. I am simply grateful that it can now be part of my lifetime plan for longevity and good health. And so should you be.

CHAPTER NINE

Estrogen: Restoring a Woman's Losses

ONE DAY IN FEBRUARY 1963, A NEW PATIENT ARRIVED IN THE office of Dr. Robert A. Wilson, a New York gynecologist. He saw nothing unusual in that, but when she said she was fifty-two, Dr. Wilson's interest level rose. He had assumed she was much younger. "Her breasts were supple and firm," he later wrote, "her carriage erect. She had good general muscle tone, no dryness of the mucuous membranes and no visible genital atrophy. Above all, her skin was smooth and pliant as a girl's."

Fifty-two-year-old women of whom such things can be said are much more usual now than they were in 1963. The reason, of course, is estrogen. Approximately 10 million postmenopausal American women are currently on the hormone, and during the remainder of this decade, as a generation of baby boomers hits their first hot flash, the number is expected to jump dramatically.

Dr. Wilson went on in 1966 to write a best-seller, *Feminine Forever*, which stimulated the first major wave of estrogen replacement. He promised women "extended youth," and though estrogen remains controversial to this day—chiefly due to fears of cancer—Dr. Wilson's promise was, in most respects, far from hollow.

IS THE CHANGE OF LIFE NECESSARY?

Between forty-five and fifty-five, age descends upon women with a suddenness for which the male life cycle offers no parallel. Yet nearly all these physical manifestations of aging are preventable or even reversable. It is not necessary for a woman's skin to lose its elasticity and begin to wrinkle. Not necessary for her vagina to shrink and become painfully dry. Not necessary for her bones to lose calcium and begin an accelerated and potentially deadly crash process of thinning—too often a prelude to shattering. Not necessary, therefore, for her shoulders to slump, her spine to curve, her carriage to lose its air of erect and youthful vitality. And not necessary for her sex drive to lessen, her moods to swing wildly, her memory to have lapses. One and all—not necessary.

Yet the fact remains that those are the normal and expected consequences of menopause, even for the woman who does not suffer devastating hot flashes, night sweats, or major depression—that is, even for the woman who has a "good" change of life.

I don't believe that I'm alarmist about the aging process. Yet I would like to suggest that those don't sound like positive additions to any woman's life. And I haven't even mentioned yet what is perhaps the most crucial dimension added to a woman's life by menopause—a greatly increased risk of heart disease. Within fifteen years after a woman's ovaries shut down, she is as much at risk for a heart attack as a man.

It would certainly seem that a strong case for estrogen (or more properly for natural hormone replacement therapy— the combined replacement of both estrogen and progesterone in their natural forms) can be made, and ought to be made, by most doctors to most women.

Yet, I enter with trepidation into this discussion of the female hormones. Long experience has taught me that American women associate the word "hormone" with the word "cancer." I don't think this association is entirely fair, but it is deeply ingrained. Properly administered, estrogen may be associated with a slightly increased risk of breast cancer, primarily because women live much longer. As for increased uterine cancer, that risk no longer seems to exist, so long as estrogen is given with a balancing amount of progesterone.

Consider that the mere fact of taking replacement hormones has been shown to extend a woman's life very significantly. The most recent of many studies observing this effect was published by Dr. Bruce Ettinger in January 1996.[1] He had followed nearly 500 women who belonged to the Kaiser Permanente health system in California. In this study, 232 women on estrogen replacement for an average of seventeen years were compared with 222 women who had used estrogen for less than one year during that same period. Their observations proved that the death rate from all causes was reduced by 44 percent in the women on estrogen.

Forty-four percent reduction in death rate from all causes is a large number. How is such a difference possible? I think that it's possible and, indeed, unsurprising. Hormone loss in the second half of life may be "natural," but it isn't healthy. That, which is I suppose, the major theme of our book, seems self-evident. Predictable hormone decline with age is an undeclared disease, and the fact that older people have always suffered it does not alter the objectivity of that judgement. Old age remains the ultimate disease, and, in my opinion, a doctor who fails to treat it is untrue to his calling. You say that it's natural for hormones to decline? Well, I say that older people have also always suffered from hardening and narrowing of the arteries. Nevertheless, no respectable physician would suggest that such cardiovascular ills should—as a perfectly natural part of aging—be left unassisted to run their deadly course.

Virtually all the evidence we currently possess demonstrates that the loss of male and female sex hormones in the second half of life is every bit as damaging to health, vigor, mental function, energy, and ultimately longevity, as the loss of growth hormone, DHEA, and melatonin—the other major endocrine hormones we've discussed. These losses are natural all right—in the worst possible sense. Nature is preparing us for our departure. If we wish to depart life later, rather than sooner, we must be willing to make adjustments to her plan.

It is not surprising, therefore, that the sudden loss of the female hormones during menopause is tremendously damaging to youthfulness. And youthfulness is not just a fancy word for sex appeal. I don't think wanting to stay young is a negative characteristic or a frivolous desire unworthy of serious adults. Not many of us want at fifty to do exactly the same things we were doing at seventeen. But we do want to pack the maximum amount of life into living. We very much want a quality of life, right up until the moment it ends.

Take a quick look at the following page, where I list the changes that occur at menopause and the advantages of hormone replacement therapy. The loss of the sex hormones constitutes a savage attack upon the functioning of the entire female body.

I think the argument for estrogen's overwhelming value to the lives of most postmenopausal women is a sound one, but even the words "increased incidence of cancer" are very emotional. The word "cancer" has hooks and barbs attached to it. It makes me uneasy, and I know it makes my patients uneasy. In the next few sections, I'm going to explain the important advantages that hormone replacement therapy offers to women—with emphasis on a combination of both estrogen and progesterone—and then, in the

The Advantages of Hormone Replacement Therapy for Postmenopausal Women

Postmenopausal Problems	*Benefits of Hormone Therapy*
Increased heart disease	Reduced risk of heart disease
Rapid increase in bone loss	Reduced rate of bone loss
Pain and stiffness in joints	Reduction or elimination of
Tiredness	all the other problems listed
Sleep disorders	in the left-hand column.
Memory lapses	
Depression	IN ADDITION:
Inability to concentrate	Reduced risk of colon cancer
Mood swings	Reduction in osteoarthritis
Hot flashes	Reduced risk of Alzheimer's
Night sweats	
Genital atrophy	
Vaginal dryness	
Decreased sexual desire	
Breast soreness and atrophy	
Dry hair	
Growth of facial hair	
Thinning, drying, and wrinkling of skin	
Stress incontinence (leakage of urine on coughing or straining)	
Constipation	
Bloated abdomen	

POTENTIAL PROBLEMS CAUSED BY HORMONE THERAPY

- Increased risk of uterine cancer, but only if estrogen is replaced without a proper balance of progesterone.
- A possible increase in the statistical risk of breast cancer, but the results of various studies are so conflicting that this is far from clear.
- Possible return of menstrual bleeding, sometimes unpredictably.
- Breast and genital tenderness and fluid retention in some women (usually only during the early months of therapy).

final section of this chapter, I'll return to a discussion of cancer and its relationship to the female hormones.

OSTEOPOROSIS AND WOMEN

Osteoporosis—bone loss—is one of the most serious health hazards a woman faces in the second half of her life. As life expectancy increases, this rather mysterious illness will have to absorb a greater and greater share of medical attention. It isn't a problem that anyone gave much thought to before the second half of this century. In a period when typical life expectancy was less than fifty years, why be concerned about thinning bones—they're only likely to pose a real peril to people over sixty. Well, most women live to be over seventy now, and more than half of them live past eighty. As further steps toward longevity are taken, most women will make it past ninety. Unless we do something about bone loss, an alarmingly high percentage of them will be in wheelchairs.

The path to osteoporosis begins in females at around age twenty when bone growth is completed. From then on, an average of one percent of bone mass (structural calcium in bones) is lost yearly. At that rate, a woman of fifty will already have lost about 30 percent of her bone and a man (because male bone loss is more gradual and starts somewhat later) about 20 percent. The situation is more serious for a woman not only because she has lost a higher percent but because she has less bone to start with.

And then menopause arrives and precipitates a veritable holocaust of bone. Generally, from ages fifty to fifty-five, women lose 3–8 percent of their bone each year. An average woman may be down to 35 to 45 percent of her original young adult bone mass by age fifty-five. Around that age, the rate of loss usually slows back to 1 percent a year. If we lived in the world of pure mathematics and theory, a woman would have no bone at all by age ninety. In the real world, the situation is grievous enough.

In the early 1990s, 24 million men and women were defined as having osteoporosis—most of them women—and this epidemic of bone disease was causing 1.2 million bone fractures a year. About 130,000 of these were women with broken necks, frequently fatal. Hip fractures caused the deaths of tens of thousands more; 20 percent of elderly adults who fracture their hips are dead within six months. By the age of seventy, almost 50 percent of women have had at least one osteoporotic fracture at an estimated cost of $7 to $10 billion annually.

Just how large a difference does estrogen and progesterone make?

Hormone Replacement = Bone Preservation

It is now well established that estrogen replacement therapy, taken as a preventive before advanced bone loss occurs, can reduce the incidence of bone fractures by approximately 50 percent. But, in this aspect of dealing with the menopause, a few medical scientists have become aware in recent years that natural progesterone is almost certainly even more effective.

To understand what happens not only in correcting bone loss but in all aspects of menopause, let's briefly consider the history and functions of estrogen and progesterone in the female body.

The Hormones of Femininity

Along with its sister hormone, progesterone, estrogen is the quintessential feminine hormone—the essential feminine accompaniment to conception and birth. Estrogen and progesterone are steroid hormones (like the major male hormone, testosterone, and also the adrenal hormones, cortisone and DHEA). In childhood, estrogen is produced by the adrenal glands. Then, at puberty, ovarian production takes over, the amount rises many-fold, and a whole host of changes takes place in a girl's body: the breasts and genitalia develop, new sweat glands emerge, a layer of fat is deposited under the skin, and pubic and axillary hair develop.

All of this activity occurs around the time of menarche, usually between eleven and fourteen years old, when a girl first begins to menstruate. This is the beginning of her fertile life as a woman, and for the next thirty to forty years she will have an ovulatory cycle designed to prepare an egg for fertilization. If that doesn't occur, she'll start over again the next month. At the beginning of each monthly cycle, estrogen causes the endometrial lining of the uterus to thicken as a preparation for fertilization. Midway through the cycle an egg is actually released by the ovary (ovulation), and, at that point, there is increased production of progesterone, the other major female hormone. Progesterone, which is also being produced in the ovaries, causes the endometrial lining to soften so that, if an egg is fertilized, it can be implanted there to form a placenta. Should pregnancy fail to occur, estrogen and progesterone levels fall during the final days of the monthly cycle, and the inner lining of the uterus is shed and expelled from the body along with some blood in a process called menstruation.

Overall production of estrogen and progesterone begin to decline during a woman's thirties, but the decline is usually not sufficient to produce early symptoms or irregularities in a woman's menstrual cycle before her mid-forties. Menopause itself is defined as the last menstrual period, and since ovarian production has been declining and menstrual cycles are generally variable and unpredictable during the final few premenopausal years, a woman isn't really sure that she has reached menopause until many months after that final menstrual period.

Menopause is an inability of the ovaries to produce any more eggs combined with a radical reduction in ovarian production of the female sex hormones. Estrogen production after menopause usually falls by approximately 66 percent. Progesterone falls correspondingly. The dramatic physical changes that we outlined earlier begin to occur.

What Happens to Your Bones?

Human bone is a continual hotbed of activity. Old or damaged bone is constantly being resorbed (dissolved) by a special class of cells called *osteoclasts*. Meanwhile, new bone is getting manufactured by the osteoclasts' good cousins, the *osteoblasts*. This Mutt 'n' Jeff team never stops working, for, contrary to the image you probably have of it, bone is active, living tissue.

So what does it mean when we say that women average a 1 percent yearly loss in bone mass over most of their adult lifetime? Clearly, the demolition team is accomplishing more work than the construction crew. Though whole chapters are written in medical textbooks analzying why, that is the bottom line. At the end of a typical year, the osteoblasts haven't been able to make quite as much bone as the osteoclasts have taken apart. Since without a skeleton you're going to have a difficult time standing up to the stresses of age, I think osteoporosis is a very real longevity issue for any human being and for women in particular.

Research has shown that the two hormones—estrogen and progesterone—that women largely lose at menopause, have contrasting effects on bone. Estrogen does not appear to aid in the formation of new bone, but it does greatly slow the tremendous increase in bone resorption that occurs after menopause—assuming, of course, that its use is begun before significant bone loss occurs. Progesterone, on the other hand, being anabolic in nature actually enhances bone strength by increasing the activity of the osteoblasts.[2] (And, as I'll explain shortly, there's also evidence that a small degree of supplemental testosterone is also power-fully supportive of osteoblast activity in women.)

John R. Lee, M.D., a pioneer in research on natural progesterone, has reported actual *reversal* of bone loss in women who combine nutritional supplementation using calcium, magnesium, and vitamins C and D together with 330 to 350 mg of transdermal natural progesterone applied to the skin in a cream. Many women in Dr. Lee's study experienced as much as a 15 percent increase in bone density over a one-year period. Women over seventy, who had already suffered significant osteoporosis with collapse of vertebrae and loss of height, improved the most.

This rate of increase in the density of weakened bone is highly unusual, and clearly more studies will be needed to confirm it. But other studies already confirm the essential and amazing fact: It is possible to reverse bone loss. A ten-year double blind study published in *Obstetrics and Gynecology* found increases in bone mass when estrogen and progesterone therapy was initiated within three years of menopause.[3]

The degree of protection from fractures is directly related to the duration of hormone use. In one study, after three to five years of replacement therapy, the likelihood of suffer-ing a fracture had declined by 11 percent. After ten years, the reduction was 50 percent. Decreased risk of hip frac-tures, wrist fractures, and spinal fractures were all observed.[4]

The evidence clearly indicates that most women don't need to go through the second half of life with curved spines and fragile, weakened skeletons. Once again, the hormones we had when young are capable of securing us a quality of physical life much closer to youth than to the conventional image of old age.

Estrogen Protects Your Mind

Research conducted in California by scientists at McGill University indicates that estrogen also helps protect women from Alzheimer's disease. The researchers studied 253 older women over several years and found that 18 percent of those who had not had estrogen therapy were subsequently diagnosed with Alzheimer's compared with 7 percent of the women who received the therapy after menopause.[5] In another study researchers examined the death certificates and the medical charts of 2,418 women who had lived in Leisure World retirement communities in southern California and had died between 1981 and 1992. Those who had been on estrogen turned out to be 40 percent less likely to have suffered Alzheimer's.[6]

Even in healthy postmenopausal women, estrogen seems to support memory. When doctors at Stanford University gave recall tests to seventy-two older women who were estrogen users (average duration of use: thirteen years) and a control group of seventy-two women of similar age and education who did not take the hormone, they found that the ability to remember names was 39 percent better among the estrogen users.[7] As we mentioned previously, this corresponds very well with the known biochemistry of the brain. Men need estrogen for proper brain function just as much as women and therefore convert testosterone to estrogen within their brains.

Probably, as we learn more about the brain, all of this will make perfect sense. Research by Dr. Bruce McEwen at Rockefeller University in New York, indicates that the steroid hormones provide potent chemical signals to the neurons in our brains even when delivered by substances not originally generated in the brain. Thus estrogen, progesterone, and testosterone—all of which are potent steroids— appear to directly affect the central nervous system, and the female hormones have been shown to influence such crucial neurotransmitters as dopamine, acetylcholine, and serotonin.

Those neurotransmitters are also significant for controlling mood and that could explain the frequency of depression in postmenopausal women.

Whatever the final conclusions may be, all the first fruits of research on estrogen and the brain indicate that it has a powerful role to play in maintaining healthy brain function.

MATTERS OF
THE HEART

It's surprising but true that when interviews and surveys are conducted among American women, almost all of them are aware of the fact that bone loss accelerates after menopause but relatively few realize that heart disease also increases rapidly. So singleminded has been the emphasis on heart disease as a male health risk that few people realize that heart attacks are the greatest single cause of female death as well. Of course, few women have heart attacks in their forties or fifties. That tends to blunt the fearfulness of this killer. A whole crop of men are dead long before sixty because of heart attacks.

Nevertheless, if longevity appeals to you—and you shouldn't be reading this book if it doesn't—and if you're a woman, you had better start thinking about the health of your heart. The extraordinary fact is that women would almost certainly be more prone to heart disease than men if it weren't for the protection given them by their hormones. After all, women have smaller blood vessels, which are consequently easier to block. That's why women catch up to men in cardiac risk so fast after menopause. Most men have been blocking their arteries since they were in their twenties. A famous series of autopsies conducted on young American soldiers who had died in battle during the Korean war found that there was already considerable evidence of atherosclerosis in the arteries of these young men with an average age of twenty.

Yet, after women go through menopause, they catch up so rapidly that by their late sixties, they are having heart attacks often as men.

Epidemiologists—medical scientists who study disease as it appears in large populations—have been conducting studies for decades now to determine if replacement of the female hormones will help protect women from heart attacks. The evidence is strongly positive. Evaluations by some of the leading epidemiologists in the country at institutions like Harvard and the University of California have reported that when all the evidence is gathered, there is a reduction in the risk of death from heart disease among women receiving hormone replacement therapy of approximately 50 percent over nonusers. In other words, if you don't take estrogen, you're twice as likely to die of a heart attack in the decades after menopause than if you do.

A metanalysis comparing thirteen leading studies done in the '70s and '80s to determine estrogen's effect on heart disease concluded that in any group of postmenopausal women on estrogen 5 percent more would die annually if they were not on the hormone.

The reason for this protective effect is quite complicated and, indeed, not completely understood, but higher levels of "good" HDL cholesterol and lower levels of "bad" LDL cholesterol are definitely part of the picture. Many studies have also found that glucose and insulin levels are lower in treated groups, and doctors have become more and more aware in recent years that high insulin levels are a significant risk factor for heart disease.

WHAT SORT OF ESTROGEN? WHAT SORT OF PROGESTERONE?

Having done what I can to make the case for replacement of the female hormones, I want to talk about what I regard as the very best program you can use. I am indebted to Dr. Jonathan Wright of Kent, Washington, who did the original research on this method of estrogen/progesterone replacement therapy. The therapy combines three kinds of estrogen with natural progesterone.

First, let's look at estrogen. In your body, estrogen is actually composed of three hormones called estrone, estradiol, and estriol. Estrone and estradiol are more commonly used in estrogen therapy because they are more potent estrogens. Unfortunately they are also more prone to promote cell growth and therefore the possibility of cancer. Estriol is a much weaker estrogen but equally effective when given in sufficient quantities. Moreover, studies have shown that estriol actually has an anti-cancer effect. In 1978 Dr. Alvin Follingstad published an article in the *Journal of the American Medical Association*, in which he proposed that estriol should became the main form of estrogen used in hormone replacement. Further reinforcement of his views came from a study in which 37 percent of women with a fast-spreading form of breast cancer experienced arrest or regression of their lesions after taking estriol.[8]

The most commonly used form of estrogen is known as *conjugated estrogens*, one of the most prescribed examples being Premarin (made, incidentally, from *preg*nant *mare*s' ur*ine*, sometimes referred to irreverantly as "horse-piss" estrogen). Unfortunately estrogen in this form is mostly converted to estradiol in the body. Wright's breakthrough was to prescribe a form of estrogen that he called tri-estrogen. Tri-estrogen is a combination capsule containing 80 percent estriol, 10 percent estrone, and 10 percent estradiol. The estrone and estradiol components are needed because in order to obtain the optimal beneficial effects of estrogen using *only* estriol, it would be necessary to give 10 to 15 mg a day, and, at that dosage, some women experience severe nausea.

In my own practice, I am now using tri-estrogen plus progesterone in total doses of either 2.5 mg or 5 mg of estrogen taken twice a day. The lower dose is equivalent to .625 mg of Premarin and the higher dose to 1.25 mg. By combining the estrogen with natural progesterone in the same capsule, further menstrual bleeding is suppressed, which eliminates the need to cycle the dosage. Because the progesterone is taken throughout the month, the action of estrogen on the lining of the endometrium is blocked, i.e., there is no build-up of the lining and therefore nothing to be sloughed off and expelled from the uterus in the manner a woman has been used to each month during menstruation. Frequently during the first few months after this replacement plan is put into place, there will be some unpredictable bleeding. Then as the lining of the uterus shrinks down and dries up due to the action of progesterone, the bleeding will stop. In virtually all cases, bleeding has stopped within six months.

Estrogen without progesterone (certainly in the conjugated estrogen form usually prescribed) has been shown quite clearly to cause precancerous cell changes in the uterus that can eventually lead to uterine cancer. This is because the buildup in the lining of the uterus that, in a normal menstrual cycle, occurs only during the first half of the month, becomes a continuous process with estrogen alone, causing excessive cellular proliferation. Add progesterone to the estrogen, however, and this effect is prevented. Many doctors cycle estrogen and progesterone during alternate parts of the month to mimic a normal menstrual cycle, but, as described above, I prefer to give progesterone throughout the month, sparing the patient the aggravation of lifelong monthly bleeding.

I believe it is much better to use natural progesterone. Most women receiving combined therapy are actually being prescribed progestins such as Provera. Such synthetic progestins have subtle chemical differences from the natural forms of the hormone, which are usually made from soybeans or wild Mexican yams.

Research seems to show that progestins do not rebuild bone as effectively as natural progesterone. The recently completed Postmenopausal Estrogen/Progestin Interventions (PEPI) Trial sponsored by the National Heart, Lung, and Blood Institute also showed that heart-protective HDL cholesterol levels were significantly higher in women using natural progesterone.[9]

Some of the Most Commonly Asked Questions About Natural Oral Progesterone

Question: What's the difference between natural and synthetic progesterone?

Answer: Progesterone, first crystallized in 1934, is available today from plant sources. Natural micronized progesterone is an exact chemical duplicate of the progesterone that is normally produced by the ovary. Synthetic progesterone, called progestins, mimic the action of progesterone, but the body does not respond in the same way, and studies have shown that progestins actually reduce the level of progesterone in the blood stream.

Question: Are there side effects with natural progesterone?

Answer: Natural progesterone is short on side effects because, unlike synthetic forms, it can make a perfect connection with progesterone receptor sites. Perhaps the only disadvantage to natural progesterone is that it is short-acting, and to maintain adequate blood levels it has to be dosed at least twice daily. A small number of women experience transient light-headedness or drowsiness.

Question: Is the oral form of natural progesterone approved by the FDA?

Answer: Natural progesterone has FDA approval. The oral form of natural progesterone is compounded from a physician's prescription by a licensed pharmacist using approved ingredients and does not require separate approval.

The reason synthetic progestins were originally developed was because, at that time, natural progesterone was not efficiently absorbed across the intestinal tract when taken orally. This is no longer a problem since micronized progesterone became available. Many hormones, including estrogen, testosterone, and DHEA are most effectively absorbed in a micronized form. That's a term for suspending microscopic particles of the hormones in an oil-filled capsule. When swallowed in this form, a portion of the progesterone is absorbed through the lymphatic system, bypassing the liver and showing increased activity in the body.

In my opinion, the combination of tri-estrogen with natural progesterone is simply the best available. Progesterone is given in 100 mg doses two times a day. The only way for you to obtain natural progesterone and tri-estrogen is to have your doctor write a prescription for it, which you can then present to a compounding pharmacy. The pharmacy I refer my patients to is the Women's International Pharmacy, Sun City West, Arizona, 1-800-279-5708.

To properly understand the so-called "sex hormones," it is important to realize that they do not relate exclusively to one sex or the other. For example, brain function is dependant on estrogen in both sexes. Men convert testosterone into estrogen in their brains.

Women also produce testosterone, in addition to estrogen. It is the ratio between male and female hormones that differs with gender—not the presence or absence of sex-specific hormones. In a young adult woman, the level of testosterone is approximately one-tenth that of a male. This relatively small amount of testosterone is extremely important for the female quality of life. Yet, after menopause, testosterone levels also fall in women. Thus women, too, experience a measure of what in men has been called andropause. Studies have shown that a woman's total estrogen production decreases by 70 to 80 percent following menopause and her testosterone production falls by about 50 percent.

Women are fearful that if they use testosterone it will cause them to grow beards and develop deep male voices, perhaps even male-pattern baldness. Well, it's true that if a woman were given a *male* dose of testosterone (especially if there were no estrogen to oppose it), she would probably experience some of those changes. (Similarly, men given high doses of estrogen will develop feminizing changes such as enlarged breasts and diminished hairiness.) If, however, the levels of both estrogen and testosterone do not exceed the normal hormonal output of a healthy woman of child-bearing age, then such problems are simply not observed.

In a recent study reported by Dr. Angela Bowen at a meeting of the North American Menopause Society, it was shown that a low dose of androgen (testosterone) given with estrogen replacement therapy was more effective than estrogen alone. In a randomized study, a number of older women were divided into two groups. One group received only estrogen, and the other group received estrogen combined with testosterone. Both treatments were well tolerated and both treatments improved the symptoms of menopause. But it was only the group whose treatment included testosterone that experienced significant relief from fatigue, insomnia, irritability, and nervousness. When treatment was stopped, benefits in the testosterone group continued for three weeks or longer. The estrogen group relapsed immediately.[10]

There is an additional, sexual factor. Testosterone promotes sexual desire in women just as it does in men, and the testosterone drop after menopause is believed to be largely responsible for the loss of sex drive that is very common in the postmenopause. A study done as far back as 1983 showed a clear correlation between the levels of testosterone that women had after menopause and their degree of sexual activity. Recent studies have shown that women who combine estrogen with testosterone in their hormone replacement therapy showed a statistical increase in sexual frequency and satisfaction compared with women who are treated with estrogen only or with nothing at all.[11]

Another Approach

There is another method of administering hormone replacement therapy about which I've received good reports from a number of sources. This involves giving estradiol and testosterone to postmenopausal women either by injection or in a pellet implanted twice yearly. Drs. C. W. Lovell (of Louisiana) and Charlton Vincente (of Missippippi) have been using this combination with great success for well over a decade. (They are also giving progesterone to their patients who still have a uterus.)

Lovell and Vincente have done a statistical analysis of four thousand of their patients on this regimen and report that the rate of breast cancer in their patients is approximately one-tenth that found in comparable age groups in the overall population. They also report an average increase of 13 percent in bone mass using estradiol and testosterone. It has been clearly demonstrated scientifically that testosterone increases osteoblast activity in bone in both men and women. Thus, a woman who has had a hysterectomy and therefore does not need progesterone for the protection of her uterus can enjoy a satisfactory formation of new bone without progesterone, if she is taking testosterone as part of her hormone replacement plan. According to Drs. Lovell and Vincente, the estradiol/testosterone combination produces improvements as well in energy, mood, libido, and sleep.

WHAT ABOUT CANCER RISK?

Finally, we come to the difficult question: will hormone replacement therapy cause cancer?

After twenty years of extensive research, the answer appears to be: Yes and No!

Here's another question: Are there any cancers HRT will protect you from? And the answer is: Probably, yes.

I wouldn't deny any woman the right to be terrified of cancer. It's a terrible disease, and anyone who has seen a loved one die of it has earned the right to be cancer phobic. But the truth is now that we combine natural progesterone with estrogen to quell the threat of precancerous growth of the endometrial tissue of the uterus, and now that we have estriol in tri-estrogen formulations available, I do not believe that the overall risk of cancer is increased, and it is probably decreased. It will take some time to do the studies needed to confirm this assumption.

Let me give you an analogy, which I certainly don't offer in an attempt to be humorous. Let's imagine that human beings had a specific incidence of cancer in their fingers. Suppose that if you lived to be a hundred with full finger function intact, you'd have a 10 percent chance of suffering finger cancer. Any way to lower that risk? Well, you could amputate a finger—or even all ten. No more finger cancer. There is, of course, a comparable analogy in the real world. One out of every three American women has had her uterus removed before the age of sixty.

In the situation that I'm imagining, there would be another approach. Let's assume that hormone replacement was necessary to maintain that full range of finger function we spoke of. Without hormones, the fingers would atrophy and have less bulk and cell mass. And let's also assume that without hormones the risk of finger cancer declines from 10 percent to 7 percent.

This is, I believe, a fairly exact description of what occurs with estrogen and breast cancer. It is not that estrogen causes cancer. Rather, it is that allowing breasts to shrink and atrophy from estrogen deficiency means there is less cell mass in which cancer can occur. Supplementing with hormones, on the other hand, maintains a normal breast, but such a breast has more and larger cells, and these cells divide more frequently to replace cells that have worn out and died. It's regrettable that this should increase cancer risk, but it may.

You don't need, of course, to maintain normal, youthful breasts to enjoy the second half of your life, but, as we've seen, you certainly can use all the other advantages, including the probability of a longer life span, which hormone replacement therapy offers you.

My program for treatment of a woman after menopause is first to ensure no history of breast cancer and, on physical examination, no evidence of breast lumps that could be malignant. If indicated, mammograms are done. Sometimes even a biopsy. To ensure uterine cancer safety, pap smears are done, and, if abnormal uterine bleeding has been present in the past, an endometrial or intrauterine sampling to rule out any hidden malignancies.

One final note to further complicate this aspect of estrogen therapy. The *Journal of the National Cancer Institute* reported in April 1995 on results from a seven-year study of estrogen use and colon cancer. They found that women who took estrogen—even though it was for less than a year—reduced their risk of dying of colon cancer by 19 percent. Women who had taken estrogen for eleven or more years were 46 percent less likely to die of the disease.[12] Scientists have speculated that estrogen lowers the concentration of bile acids, thereby creating an environment hostile to the growth of cancer cells in the colon. Another theory has it that estrogen directly suppresses tumor growth in the lining of the colon. Either way, the effect on women's life expectancy is significant, since after the breast and lungs, colon cancer is the third highest killer cancer in women.

So, there is evidence that estrogen actually prevents cancer.

One final point about cancer. Preventing it can only be done with the aid of a full program of healthy living. When percentages are given for the number of people who are going to get breast cancer or prostate cancer or any other common malignancy, those figures are based on a population that contains very sizable numbers of people who do not eat properly, who do not take supplemental vitamins and minerals, who do not exercise, and who smoke or drink too much. Their risks are much different from yours, if you're a person who's seriously trying for a long and healthy life. Look carefully at Chapters Thirteen and Fourteen, in which we talk about an ideal diet and supplemental nutrition program.

CONCLUSION

In spite of the abundant advantages of hormone replacement therapy, I know that the estrogen choice remains a tough one for many women. They wonder how great the breast cancer risk is, they wonder whether the expectation of increased longevity is really as soundly based as it appears to be. A totally definitive answer cannot be given at this time, but the evidence I've given above is not only quite convincing but supported by a lot of research.

In 1994 the National Institutes of Health launched the $628 million Women's Health Initiative research study. One part of that research project will involve 27,500 women, half of them randomly assigned to receive HRT, the other half a placebo. Scientists will track the women for at least eight years comparing heart disease, osteoporosis, and breast cancer rates in the two groups. Unfortunately a final report isn't expected to be ready before 2005. None of the women in that study will receive estrogen in the form of estriol, and none will receive natural progesterone.

Therefore, the results will not fully apply to the regimen I'm recommending, but unless this research project is in startling contradiction to studies that have been done in the past, we will see an impressive reconfirmation of the life-extending effects of hormone replacement with the female sex hormones.

CHAPTER TEN

The Male Andropause and Testosterone Replacement

WHY AREN'T MEN TAKING THE SAME SORT OF HORMONE replacement that women are? Why isn't testosterone the treatment of choice for the aging male? Many physicians practicing today are beginning to conclude that an eventual surge of male hormone replacement is the only logical approach to the health needs of the older male.

Of course, there are many psychological, historical, and societal reasons why it hasn't happened yet, including, I'm quite sure, a macho reluctance on the part of many men to concede the possibility of their sex hormone production being in any way inadequate.

There's a crystal clear biological reason, too: A man's level of testosterone doesn't suddenly fall off the edge of the table the way a menopausal woman's estrogen and progesterone levels do. There's no screaming emergency in the hormone department, no hot flashes, no alarming decline in bone, no sudden genital atrophy. Men can pretend nothing is happening to them.

All the same, it is.

By the time they reach their seventies, most men have 30 to 50 percent less testosterone than they had when young. This clearly has an effect on their sex drive, which we'll explore in a moment. But, if you're a man, be aware that it weakens you in many other ways as well. Together with the decline in growth hormone, testosterone's drop shares responsibility for the loss of muscle mass and the subsequent erosion of strength. There's evidence as well that the testosterone dip contributes to loss of bone. Of even more significance for your basic survival, there have been striking studies done in the past five years that have shown that lower testosterone levels correlate with *increased* risk for heart disease—exactly the opposite of what doctors used to imagine the male hormone's cardio-vascular effects were. It was almost a cliché, you know: poor men, their sex hormones kill them. In fact, nothing could be further from the truth.

Finally, there is a correlation between loss of testos-terone and a generalized loss of functionality. Eugene Shippen, M.D., one of the most experienced doctors I know in this field, reports that every man in his eighties or nineties who he treats and who's still physically and men-tally vigorous has high normal testosterone levels for his age. *He's never seen an exception!*

Perhaps it makes sense to start testosterone supple-mentation as one gets older. I wonder.

ISN'T THIS A BIG, BAD STEROID?

Before we go any further, it's best to admit that testos-terone has a terrible reputation. It is, after all, the princi-pal anabolic steroid in the human body. The exact name is androgenic-anabolic steroid, and we get that term from the two Greek words *andro* and *gennan*, meaning "male-producing," and from another Greek word, *anabold*, meaning "to build up." And some men (and a few women) certainly do get built up. We all have images of overdeveloped and overambitious athletes taking illegal steroids on the q.t. to gain an edge, their biceps bulging like melons about ready to pop through the tightly stretched, fat-free flesh of their arms. The consequences for their health are serious. Unnatural levels of steroid hormones can cause sterility, coronary artery disease, serious liver damage, and brain tumors. The latter was what Lyle Alzado, the All-Pro defensive lineman for the Los Angeles Raiders and an admitted steroid abuser, died of.

So steroids are dangerous? Absolutely, but slow down and consider what we mean here. Steroids taken at levels the human body was never meant to handle are exceedingly dangerous. Young men and women have no business taking artificial steroids. They are already enjoying their natural maximum levels of testosterone. Assuming your glands were functioning normally when you were in your twenties, you can be quite certain that the level of testosterone you had then was the highest nature intended you to have: your natural max. As a result, the average twenty-year-old male who wants to get athletic is usually going to find himself building a fairly formidable set of muscles simply with the aid of natural exertion. Young women can create smaller but highly efficient musculature if they want to, too.

At this point, let me reiterate something that was thoroughly discussed in Chapter Nine for any of you who skipped that chapter. Testosterone is not exclusively a male hormone. Women secrete testosterone at about one-tenth the level of their male counterparts. And their testosterone is exceedingly important to them just as it is to the male half of the human race. In fact, many doctors are now beginning to add small amounts of testosterone to the estrogen and progesterone replacement plan that they prescribe for their postmenopausal female patients. The results are excellent. So go back to Chapter Nine for details, if you're a woman. The rest of this chapter is going to concentrate on the men. For them, testosterone may be both life-saving and life-enhancing.

Let's return to what this chapter, and indeed this book, is about—that is, hormone replacement therapy, *not* self-induced hormone overdoses. There is no evidence at all to suggest that testosterone supplementation to replace the amounts lost as the result of aging can cause damage to the male body. All the evidence shows the exact contrary. So, in reading the rest of this chapter, put out of your mind those frightening images of beefed-up, overly aggressive football players damaging their health and breaking the law to further their careers. Hundreds of thousands of men are, indeed, doing that—including teenage boys. One study reports that 7 percent of male high school seniors have taken anabolic steroids. This is potentially tragic, but it has nothing to do with the subject of this chapter. Like human growth hormone, testosterone is a natural hormone that promotes cell growth, protein synthesis, and healing. Because it's a very special hormone—a sex hormone—it also in some measure promotes sexual vigor. These are desirable objectives, and they can be best obtained by maintaining the normal and not by supplementing into the range of the abnormal.

What Happens to Men?

Why do so many men feel despair and decline in their fifties and early sixties? A masculine tradition of "keeping it all in" has throttled open discussion of this phenomenon. At best there are rather vague and patronizing references to a "midlife crisis," but nobody seems to know just what that is or why it should be happening. The male andropause is a hidden pause; it's nothing like the perfectly evident transition that a woman in her early fifties is experiencing. Neither hot flashes like blow torches, nor the complete cessation of entire biological systems.

Yet many men—and doctors know this—are experiencing a deep grinding desperation in this period of their life. I've seen men come close to suicide, only to recover when something was done about their hormones. Sexual malaise is an obvious element. Most men begin to experience at least some reduction in desire, in frequency of erections, in overall sexual function in their forties. Whether all this change is due to testosterone decline is not entirely clear, but there is little doubt that much of it is. Testosterone has a very direct influence on sexuality. Younger men who have uncharacteristically low hormonal levels generally have low sex drives, but they will display increased sexual interest and activity if given testosterone replacement. The reverse effect occurs when drugs designed to suppress testosterone are given to men suffering from prostate cancer. Impotence usually results. There are reports that indicate that there is a testosterone threshold—which varies considerably from person to person—below which sexual function is impaired.

Of course, though testosterone declines steadily with age, many if not most men remain sexually potent right into old age. It is not impotence so much as a declining interest and enthusiasm that usually occurs. How burdensome that will be depends on the personality of the individual male.

It would seem that the loss of enthusiasm for life that afflicts many men in middle age is a combination of a number of factors. The physical factors—declining sexual vigor and diminished strength, energy, and muscle mass—are closely related to the slipping level of testosterone. Some mental and psychological symptoms may also be the result of this slippage. The mental energy and excitability of youth can fall off very sharply as testosterone declines. That high testosterone levels are partly responsible for that energy is certainly indicated by the fact that many men recover their creativity and drive after testosterone replacement therapy. You probably remember my mentioning in the previous chapter that estrogen is the steroid hormone of most significance to brain function and that in men testosterone is chemically reformulated into estrogen in the brain. Without proper levels of testosterone that is clearly hard to do.

Testosterone is a hormone of marvelous versatility. Like the other anti-aging hormones we've discussed, its effects are widespread in the body and far from limited to what one might expect from a "sex" hormone. Dr. Richard S. Wilkinson has related the following case.

One of his patients, a wealthy research physicist, started experiencing physical problems in his late forties—allergies and a back problem came first. A general sense of being "run-down" followed in the succeeding years. At fifty-five, a severe heart irregularity was added to the list. The physicist turned to the world famous Scripps Clinic in southern California, but an extensive workup (at a cost I shudder to contemplate) found nothing to explain his growing debilitation. Pressed by their patient, who was neither personally nor scientifically inclined to accept easy answers, they could only suggest that perhaps he was "aging a little faster than normal."

I need hardly say that that workup did not include checking his blood testosterone levels. The physicist decided to seek his own answers. He wondered why his energy was so low and why so many parts of his body seemed incapable of working well more or less simultaneously. Being professionally knowledgeable about feedback mechanisms, his interest turned toward the endocrine hormones, clearly one of the body's main feedback control systems.

Eventually he found a physician who was willing to work with him in investigating his hormones. They quickly scored two bullseyes. The wealthy physicist proved to have both low thyroid function and a low testosterone level—

either one of these would have been sufficient to account for his fatigue. The story, of course, has a happy ending. Thyroid therapy and testosterone replacement returned the patient to virtually the man he had been ten years before. I've seen stories like this end sadly. I suspect the right approach not only rejuvenated the physicist but perhaps saved him from an early death.

Testosterone has to be taken seriously. It's not just an essential part of your sex life or a dubious muscle aid for foolhardy athletes. Let's look at the history of this hormonal treatment.

SOME VERY ODD ATTEMPTS

The idea of restoring the male sex hormones as a means of rejuvenation is not a new one. Indeed, its history is long, colorful, and somewhat bizarre.[1]

The forefather of testosterone replacement therapy was undoubtedly Charles Edouard Brown-Sequard, a prominent French professor of physiology, who announced on June 1, 1889, that he had discovered a rejuvenating therapy. The seventy-two-year-old scientist believed that he had reversed his own decline by injecting himself with a liquid extract derived from the testicles of dogs and guinea pigs. These injections, he told his audience at the Societé de Biologie in Paris, had radically increased his physical strength and intellectual energy, as well as lengthening the arc of his urine.

Today virtually everyone agrees that the improvements Brown-Sequard observed were due to the power of suggestion. Nonetheless, the aging physiologist had revived in a more sophisticated form ideas that have a long history in human culture and popular medicine. The ancient Egyptians had attributed medicinal value to the testicles, and the Roman naturalist, Pliny the Elder, reported that the oil-soaked penis of a donkey and the honey-coated penis of a hyena were used as sexual fetishes. Medical authorities in ancient India had recommended the ingestion of testis tissue as a cure for impotence. A German compendium of remedies published in 1754 mentions the use of horse testicles and the sexual parts of marine animals as aphrodisiacs.

Putting to one side the obvious element of wishful thinking in these "therapies," there is perhaps in all of them a vague insight into the possibility that the functions of the testicles might be restored by finding some replacement for the substances they produce.

Another approach was an actual testicle transplant, and this extraordinary notion actually met with some success. In 1912, two physicians in Philadelphia transplanted a testicle into a patient. Apparently the surgery was successful, but reports of its long-term effects have not survived. A year later in Chicago, Dr. Victor Lespinasse removed a testicle from a donor, fashioned it into three transverse slices, and inserted them into a sexually dysfunctional patient who had lost both his own testicles. The man felt so invigorated sexually that within a matter of days, he stormed out of the hospital in search of satisfaction. Lespinasse reported that two years later the man's sexual function was still intact.

Further efforts were made by Dr. Leo L. Stanley, resident physician at San Quentin prison in California. Starting in 1918, he began transplanting testicles from recently executed prisoners into inmates, some of whom reported the recovery of sexual potency. Stymied by the "scarcity of human material," Stanley went on to transplant the testes of rams, goats, deer, and boars into men with some reported success. This dubious approach was soon followed by the Russian-French surgeon Serge Voronoff, who made a fortune in the 1920s with his controversial "monkey gland" transplants. This line of treatment soon acquired an unfortunate aura of quackery that still hangs over the whole subject of male hormone replacement.

The abuse of steroids for muscle building and the fear that testosterone, if given to women, would result in virilizing side effects such as deeper voices and hirsutism were not helpful either.

Nonetheless, for a moment in the 1930s and 1940s, it seemed that testosterone therapy might take off. The necessary scientific foundation for real testosterone replacement was laid in 1935 when Dutch doctors isolated testosterone and created a synthetic form of it for the first time. Doctors began using it in men with hypogonadism—that's medicalese for levels of testosterone so low as to prevent normal sexual development. Soon older men whose testosterone decline had caused impotence were also being treated. Such uses are still regarded as medically sound.

What didn't happen for men, however, was what has occurred with postmenopausal women since the 1950s—a full-scale program of hormone replacement essentially designed to counteract aging. Only in the 1990s has it become apparent that this is both a logical—and perhaps inevitable—next step.

TESTOSTERONE PROTECTS HEALTH

In the last seven or eight years, scientific interest in the male hormone has come alive. Studies have been conducted on men in their middle years or older who have low or normal testosterone levels for their age range. Almost invariably, the results have been positive. Men have gained muscle and consequent strength, there have been indications of a slowdown in bone resorption (the process of bone loss), there has been increase in sexual desire and functionality, and studies have shown better spatial cognition and word memory.

Does all this have an impact on longevity? Does testosterone deserve to be regarded as one of the pro-longevity hormones? I don't have any doubt that eventually it will be seen as one of the most powerful of them, especially in males. Let's be very practical for a moment. We all know that heart disease eventually ends the life of the majority of American males. How does testosterone relate to this?

Its original imagined relationship was by way of a bit of popular mythology. Doctors, I've found, are as prone to simplistic thinking as anyone else. Therefore, they didn't object when in a classic of faulty logic, the following syllogism was constructed: "Males have most of the heart attacks and males have most of the testosterone, therefore testosterone causes heart attacks." Only, it ain't so. A long string of studies has demonstrated the opposite. Consider a few of the most recent.

Dr. Gerald Philips's team at the Columbia University College of Physicians and Surgeons followed fifty-five men with chest pain or other signs of atherosclerotic heart disease and set about measuring their levels of testosterone. Then they took angiograms (pictures of their coronary arteries) and found that there was a clear correlation. The men with low levels of testosterone were far more likely to have significantly clogged arteries than the men with high levels. Moreover, the men with low testosterone levels had higher levels of such cardiovascular risk factors as fibrinogen and insulin and lower levels of heart-protective HDH (good) cholesterol.[2]

These are fairly convincing indications that testosterone is heart protective. Here are three other studies. In one, Swedish researchers gave testosterone for eight months to twenty-three middle-aged men. The men's blood sugar, diastolic blood pressure, and cholesterol all went down, and their insulin resistance improved.[3] In another study, Dr. Joyce Tenover of the University of Washington gave testosterone to thirteen men whose natural levels were low and their muscle mass increased and both their total cholesterol and their LDL ("bad") cholesterol went down.[4] These men randomly received injections of either testosterone or a placebo for three months. Dr. Tenover reports that twelve of the thirteen men knew without being told in which period they were receiving testosterone because they became aware of an increase in their sex drive, in their assertiveness in business dealings, and because of an improvement in energy level and general sense of well-being.

The final study is significant because of its relatively greater size. Epidemiologists at Vanderbilt University Medical Center examined the records of the Caerphilly Heart Disease Study, which followed 2,512 men in Wales between 1978 and 1982. Those who developed heart disease were found to have had significantly lower testosterone levels than their healthier brethren. Most heart protective indicators, including levels of good HDL cholesterol, were higher in the high-testosterone males.[5]

TESTOSTERONE RESTORES VITALITY

And what if you're already old and somewhat tired? Can testosterone make a major difference? Although in my own practice, I usually combine testosterone replacement therapy with many of the other pro-longevity hormones you've already read about, I've also talked to doctors whose speciality is testosterone. They report remarkable examples of relative rejuvenation from testosterone alone.

Dr. Eugene Shippen had an eighty-three-year-old patient named Jasper Saloway, who was recently widowed. At first, Jasper was severely depressed, but eventually he acquired a woman friend and began a romantic relationship. His depression went away, and his mood and functioning seemed excellent. But then, in the following year, he started going through a decline. He had headaches and dizzy spells, and his sex function declined. Dr. Shippen measured his testosterone level and found it was very low—around 150—very far from the desirable range of 500 to 800 ng/dl. He persuaded him to start taking testosterone, and around six weeks later Jasper came in for a review. His symptoms had gotten markedly better, and his energy level was much higher.

"But what about sex, Jasper?" Dr. Shippen asked.

"Oh, that—I got an erection you could have hung a paint bucket on."

We've already mentioned that testosterone can have positive effects on mental functioning. Another one of Dr. Shippen's patients was a dramatic example.

Charlie McCormick was a retired lawyer, eighty-five years old and happily married for more than fifty years. He gave every indication of someone who was becoming senile. He had been going downhill in energy and zest for a couple of years, but now when he came with his wife to see Dr. Shippen, the prognosis looked pretty grim. He sat slumped in his chair, not speaking, and didn't seem able to understand the questions that the doctor was asking him. Eventually Dr. Shippen had to get all the answers from Charlie's wife, and when Charlie left the room to have his blood drawn, she told him that he was like this almost all the time now. To Dr. Shippen this looked as if it were the early stages of Alzheimer's or else severe atherosclerosis affecting the oxygen supply to the brain. But under the circumstances and looking at the low testosterone on Charlie's blood test, he decided to gamble on its being hormonal shortages. With some difficulty, he convinced the McCormicks to try testosterone and come back to see him again in a few weeks.

When they did, Charlie looked more energetic, but, more importantly, he was able to understand all the questions that Dr. Shippen asked him. At another visit a few weeks later, the improvement was still more evident. Charlie was telling jokes and holding up his end of a reasonable conversation. Charle's wife told the good doctor that he was a miracle worker. That was two years ago and since then Charlie—still on testosterone—has been feisty, functioning, and essentially back to normal.

It is simply a fact, which I have seen repeatedly in clinical practice, that a significant percentage of older people who seem to be failing have nothing seriously wrong with them except a correctable shortage of hormones—almost always the hormones we're writing about in this book.

WHO NEEDS TESTOSTERONE?

In a young man, testosterone levels will generally be between 800 and 1100 nanograms per deciliter (ng/dl). As men age, this goes down quite unpredictably. There are seventy-year-olds whose testosterone will be as high as 700, and others who will be at 200 or even lower. In my experience—and many doctors I've spoken to quote numbers not far different from this—a man with low blood levels of testosterone will experience a satisfying improvement in his energy and general well-being if he takes replacement doses that bring his levels into the 500 to 800 range. There does not seem to be any reason to aim for the high end of the youthful scale.

If a man has been experiencing loss of sexual interest or occasional impotence, testosterone replacement can sometimes result in dramatic improvement. And some doctors have noted that a testosterone cream placed directly on the penis can help with erectile difficulties. But do remember that testosterone is not a cure-all. There are serious sexual problems that are not testosterone related. Impotence can result from advanced atherosclerosis that has severely

The PSA Dilemma

Men are rightly fearful of prostate cancer, now the second highest killer cancer in males, and this sometimes makes them hesitant to embrace testosterone replacement. The prostate, a gland about the size of a walnut, makes the liquid portion of semen, tends to enlarge with age, and frequently becomes cancerous. It is usually a slow-growing cancer, and autopsies have shown that one out of three men who die over the age of eighty from other causes had prostate cancer without knowing it.

In the last decade, a test for a substance in the blood called prostate-specific antigen (PSA) has been refined sufficiently to give doctors a real shot at diagnosing prostate cancer without biopsying the organ. It's usually considered—all other things being equal—that a middle-aged man with a PSA over 4 has some possibility of cancer; if the PSA is over 10, the indication is quite strong, and a biopsy will be performed. Men with enlarged prostates or prostate infections (prostatitis) can have prostates in the 4–10 range and be quite free of cancer, so it's useful to estimate the size of the prostate and do a PSA/volume ratio in order to avoid unnecessary biopsies.

The relationship of all this to testosterone is quite simple. There is no evidence that testosterone will produce cancer cells in the prostate if there are none there, but it will stimulate cancer-cell growth that has already begun.

Thus, testosterone replacement therapy should always be accompanied in any man over forty with regular—preferably twice yearly—PSA tests and a yearly manual prostate exam. Because of this precaution, we can say that testosterone, far from being a cause of prostate cancer, will help to act as an early warning system. If any suspicion of prostate cancer does arise, a decision will almost certainly be made to stop testosterone therapy.

weakened the blood supply to the penis (heavy smokers are particularly subject to this); from extreme obesity; and from diabetes, which sometimes damages the blood vessels and nerves in the penis.

Administration

Testosterone can be administered through an unusual range of methods, and many doctors are vigorous advocates of different modes of administration. The one thing that can be said for certain is that oral administration of the natural form is poorly absorbed. Most oral testosterones go through the portal vein from the intestine to the liver and the liver inactivates a sizable percentage of the hormone. Some of this loss can be avoided by using the micronized form of testosterone suspended in oil. Some of that bypasses the liver and is absorbed by the lymphatic system, but, in my experience, such testosterone stays in the body for only an hour or two, and the effects rapidly fade. There are synthetic forms of testosterone—such as methyl-testosterone—which are well absorbed by mouth, with a long half-life, but I strongly advise against using them since there are reliable reports associating them with cancer of the liver.

Of the remaining methods of administration, I usually advise either injections or the use of creams and gels that are absorbed through the skin. The long-acting injectable testosterone comes in two forms—enanthate and cypionate—both are in thick, viscous solutions to prolong their action. Once injected, the testosterone is slowly released into the body over a three-week period, and during that time a relatively steady level of testosterone is maintained in the body. Between 100 and 200 mg are injected every two to three weeks. Blood levels are monitored. I think the concentration that's achieved in this way is closer to the levels found in young men than what can be obtained with creams and gels. However, because of the thickness of the solution, a testosterone injection requires a relatively large needle, and some men are not enthusiastic.

Fortunately, creams and gels also work well, if applied daily on schedule. In fact, Dr. Eugene Shippen favors them over injections, because he believes the more variable levels they cause are a better copy of what the body does on its own. Your body produces the lion's share of its testosterone during the nighttime hours—which is why young men so often wake with erections—and by applying a cream or a gel just before bedtime, a similar effect can be achieved. The cream is rubbed into the thin skin of the scrotum or inside the thighs where absorption is best. The gel can be used anywhere but usually not on the scrotum since this causes many men to experience a burning sensation. If your pharmacy has the testosterone imbedded in a patch, you may opt for this mode, which is a little bit neater. Some men, however, will find that a patch can cause skin irritation. If you don't use a patch, the testosterone cream or gel should be well rubbed in.

There is yet another method of receiving testosterone. Drs. C. W. Lovell and Charlton Vincente have treated thousands of patients using pellets implanted in the buttocks once every six months. This method delivers a constant blood level of testosterone over a long period. Clearly, for maintaining a youthful testosterone profile, it's an excellent approach. There is, however, the inconvenience of a minor surgical procedure twice yearly. The cost of the procedure is not unreasonable.

All these methods are valid approaches to replacing testosterone, and I think men who are over fifty and whose blood levels of testosterone are below 400 should seriously consider such a replacement plan. The female menopause has become a standard subject for medical treatment. The less well defined male pause—the andropause—is certainly medically treatable, too. In my opinion, we men deserve no less.

PART II

The Road to Health and Longevity

CHAPTER ELEVEN

Be Aware of Your Own Individuality

I THINK IT WOULD BE VERY PLEASANT TO REACH A HUNDRED AND ten or so, reasonably fit and still mentally alert. Lots of interesting things would happen in the world while I'm watching, and I'd get to see my great-grandchildren grow up. The difference between me and many other people my age is that—for reasons that are becoming apparent—I think I have a decent chance of making it there. And I think that most of you—if you want it—have a decent chance, too.

The first thing you've all learned reading the first half of this book is that we've firmly and finally broken the back of one of the main causes of aging. We've done it in just the last ten years while nobody was looking. You no longer need to become a dried-up old prune with hardly any hormones. What a relief!

Having conquered that obstacle—and it seems incredible to think it was done so easily—let's see how many other steps we can take toward longevity. But before I outline just what the remainder of this book will dwell on, I'd like you to face up to your own individuality. Pluses and minuses!

You are:

Male or female
Fat or thin or in-between
Physically fit or somewhat less than fit

You have:

A precise age
A family background including common illnesses, which
    have felled your parents or grandparents
A personal medical history

You feel:

Healthy or somewhat sickly
Energetic or average or perhaps quite tired
Younger than your calendar years or perhaps somewhat
    older

I'm going to assume that most of you—and that probably includes you personally—have at least a few weaknesses in those areas. Most of us aren't physically perfect, nor were our ancestors. The truth is, however, that barring calamitous medical misfortunes, you can take the body and the mind you now possess and form them into a superb tool for survival. In the following chapters, I'm going to outline fairly briefly a plan of attack.

Meanwhile, if you were just like everybody else, how long would you live?

Table 11.1 tells you what a life insurance salesman knows when you mention your age.

Those tables show an actuarial expectation of life at birth of almost seventy-two years for men and somewhat less than seventy-nine for women. I'm encouraging you to aim a lot higher. After all, those tables reflect not only the longevity of average people but the rather poor longevity of tens of millions of people who smoke or drink too much or

Table 11.1
Life Expectancy

Age Range	Average Years of Life Remaining for a Male in This Age Range	Average Years of Life Remaining for a Female in This Age Range
0–1	71.8	78.6
1–5	71.6	78.3
5–10	67.8	74.4
10–15	62.8	69.5
15–20	57.9	64.6
20–25	53.3	59.7
25–30	48.7	54.9
30–35	44.1	50.1
35–40	39.6	45.3
40–45	35.1	40.5
45–50	30.7	35.8
50–55	26.4	31.3
55–60	22.3	26.9
60–65	18.6	22.7
65–70	15.2	18.8
70–75	12.1	15.2
75–80	9.4	11.9
80–85	7.1	9.0
85 and over	5.3	6.6

SOURCE: National Center for Health Statistics

take drugs or completely neglect their physical fitness through lack of exercise. Those of you who avoid those physically destructive habits are going to add many years to your life.

If, in addition, to taking sufficient exercise, you eat an exceptionally healthy diet and take nutritional supplements, you will be vastly lowering your likelihood of dying from heart disease, stroke, diabetes, and cancer.

Some people are already taking these measures, and, in combination with the development of vaccines and antibiotics in the first half of this century and other medical advances, including improved surgical techniques and improved emergency room procedures in the second half, we are seeing—indeed, we have seen—significant changes. In 1900 the average expectation of life at birth in the United States was approximately fifty years. That low level was partly due to high infant mortality and the dangers to women of childbirth. But the progress since has still been remarkable.

Moreover, the number of centenarians is steadily increasing.

Census Bureau data indicates that centenarians are among the fastest growing groups in the country. By their estimates, the population aged eighty-five and over will grow sixfold between 1980 and 2080, but the population of centenarians will grow seventy-five-fold! And they haven't taken into account yet the changes outlined in this book. In fact, so rapid is the alteration in U.S. demographics that between 1950 and 1990 the number of Americans who were a hundred or older went up by ten times. By 1990 there were 37,000 centenarians in the United States. Of course, in a country of more than 250 million people that still makes them a rare breed. But I think you can see the kinds of changes we have ahead of us.

Now, since quality of life is paramount in forming any satisfying plan for longevity, look at Table 11.2 and consider for a moment the kinds of chronic diseases most likely to afflict older people.

There's certainly a fair amount of discomfort and disability locked up in those cold statistics. Also a good deal of probable death represented by the more serious items on that list.

Yet, we know that the life-threatening problems such a list implies can be altered in the vast majority of men and women who, if they do nothing but sit back to await their fate, will certainly in the end be visited with them. Even if

Table 11.2

Percentage of People Over Age Sixty-Five with Various Chronic Conditions According to the National Center for Health Statistics

Condition	*Percent Men*	*Percent Women*
Arthritis	36	55
Hearing impairment	36	25
Hypertension	35	46
Heart disease	33	29
Limb deformity	14	19
Cataracts	10	21
Visual impairment	10	9
Emphysema	8	2
Cerebrovascular disease	8	5
Ulcers	4	3
Glaucoma	3	4
Frequent constipation	3	7
Gastritis	1	3

your own family history and the conclusions reached by your doctors when they look at your medical charts indicate, for instance, that you are a very likely candidate for heart disease—and probably sooner, rather than later—there are steps you can take. You certainly can, and should, set about fashioning a diet that will normalize your blood pressure and sharply reduce the likelihood of further free radical damage to your cardiovascular system. I call that an Anti-Free Radical Diet, as you'll see. You can start a vigorous program of nutritional supplementation. The evidence that this very significantly lowers rates of heart disease is now in. Only medical Neanderthals continue to deny it. You can have yourself treated with chelation therapy, an important though still often misunderstood therapy, that I've written about in the past. If you know nothing about it, see Appendix Two. You can develop an exercise program for yourself. I'll explain that, too. There is seldom a person so sick that he or she can't benefit from an intelligent and prudently planned program of increased exertion. You can also—depending on your financial resources and the judgment of your doctor—begin a replacement program of human growth hormone. I think I've said enough in Part One to convince most of you that that mighty muscle called your heart is particularly responsive to the repair and maintenance effects of HGH. You can do replacement therapy with DHEA. You can maintin your melatonin levels. And finally, depending on your sex, you can turn to testosterone or estrogen and progesterone for further hormonal defense against cardiovascular ills.

This is a powerful toolbox I've just described. I can't easily overemphasize the difference in life extension and in joy of life between a person who takes all these tools out and uses them for all they're worth and a person who does nothing or only one or two things to protect himself. It's easy to let life slip along assuming the best. Because there's a sort of self-selection factor involved in reading a book like this, I feel comfortable addressing the readers of this book as people who don't want to do that.

In the remainder of this book, I'm going to touch on diet, nutritional supplementation, chelation therapy, exercise, and finally how you can combine the best of these approaches with your own personal hormone replacement program. I believe that most of you have the potential to become survival superstars—and it will be a survival bristling with vigor. It will be a survival that will astonish most of your contemporaries, because—unless they learn to take a similar approach to their aging bodies—as the years pass, they will not be able to keep up with you.

Indeed, it hardly needs saying that unless they, too, replace the hormones that the years will deprive them of, their physical and mental abilities will slowly begin to fade. Systems of their bodies that are fully capable of functioning efficiently for more than a hundred years will begin to shut down, thirsting for hormones that they can never have again. But as you and I have seen, those hormones are yours for the asking. I can hardly imagine a more delightful discovery. It fills me with hope. And hope, and a resolution to continue, is what I hope to fill all of you with, too.

CHAPTER TWELVE

The Basic Joy of Exercise

EXERCISE SHOULDN'T DETAIN US FOR VERY LONG. YOU'VE HEARD
ad nauseam that it's good for you. All right, here goes
again: *It's good for you!*

The human body was meant to move. All those precise
joints, those muscles, those tendons—it's a waste of a great
structural design to leave them prone on the sofa in front
of the television set.

I don't propose to convince you that you should strive
for athletic stardom. Any Olympic gold medal winners
reading this book will undoubtedly skip this chapter. The
rest of us should set our sights on modest but constructive
goals. If I can convince all of you to build half an hour of
moderately vigorous exertion into your daily schedule, I
will have done my good deed for the month.

Once you get started, many of you won't want to stop
there. After all, as a general rule, moving the body is fun.
If you have the time and the desire you might want to double or triple the amount of exercise you get each day. The
important thing to realize is that some exercise—even fast

walking—is an essential part of a good longevity plan. The no-exercise plan—sofa to driver's seat—that so many Americans have embraced is an actively inactive abuse of the body you were born with. It's deadly for health and deprives you of much of the joy of living. So let's look at some gentle alternatives.

HOW TO BEGIN

Basically one begins by doing a little bit more than one's doing already. If you walk ten minutes a day, start walking fifteen. In a week or two, go up to twenty. If you always walk slowly, walk a little more quickly. Park the car at the far end of the parking lot by preference. Try walking up a few flights of stairs sometimes instead of taking the elevator. After a month or two of exercising more, you'll find that it's easier.

There is no question that habitual lifelong exercise is a plus. It helps burn off fat, suppresses appetite, aids circulation, improves the HDL/LDL ("good" guy/"bad" guy) ratio in serum cholesterol, reduces depression and anxiety, and, of course, increases general fitness. Exercise will make you look better and feel better, and when done with a sensible respect for your own limitations, it will eventually raise your general energy level. Incidentally, exercise also increases your body's own production of human growth hormone. You'll get some hormone replacement for free.

I am writing this chapter particularly to speak to those of you who are exercise-phobic. We live in a society full of energy-saving devices. Not too many of us are vigorous walkers anymore. The automobile has seen to that. The television set glues our posteriors down, and desk jobs restrict all too many of us to an exercise plan that involves strolling to the photocopier and the coffee cart six or seven times a day.

If this picture describes you, you've grown unused to using your muscles and you may have compromised your cardiovascular system. I want you to start slowly. Anyone past his or her mid-thirties shouldn't rush boldly into training for a marathon or playing three sets of tennis on a hot summer day. At least one study has shown that half of sudden death attacks were immediately preceded by severe or moderate exercise. Listen to your body. When it complains, slow down, rest.

Nonetheless, a slow increase of exercise is likely to pay off with many extra years of life. Coronary artery disease has been shown to be three times more prevalent among sedentary postal clerks in Washington, D.C., than among the capital's physically active mail carriers. Research in North Dakota found that non-farmers were twice as likely to have a heart attack than farmers.

For most of you, walking really will be the best way to begin. Expand your range daily and increase your speed gradually. Unless you're in very poor physical condition, you should be able to walk a mile in thirty minutes after a few weeks of practice. I hope and expect that many of you will find it so pleasant that soon you'll be walking two miles. To liven this activity up, you might want to get a dog or go to musuems and art galleries. Some people like walking in malls. (But don't blame me when the credit card bills come due.)

Your next step might be to move on to what Dr. Thomas W. Patrick, Jr., refers to as "wogging." That's simply, as the name implies, halfway between a walk and a run. If your knees, back, or ankles start to bother you, stay with the fast walk.

Many of you may decide to take up some sport or join an exercise program. Consider what is likely to attract you in the exercises described below.

THE TYPES OF EXERCISE

Aerobic Exercise

Aerobic exercise challenges your heart rate and causes increased oxygen consumption. Because the exertion level is so low, walking is only mildly aerobic. If you want to reach a higher level of fitness, consider such activities as cross-country skiing, running, swimming, rowing, bicycling, or aerobic dancing. If you're going to take up some form of vigorous aerobic exercise, you might want to get professional advice or at least purchase a self-help book related to the type of exercise you plan to do. You'll be able to learn limbering and stretching exercises to help prevent injuries to your muscles and joints. Perhaps you'll need special shoes. Running, because of its impact on your knees and ankles, requires special care. Don't rush into any of this if you're significantly overweight. See if you can get some of the weight off first to minimize the possibility of injuring your joints. With all exercises other than walking, it's probably best to warm up slowly and do stretching exercises first, unless you're exceptionally limber.

Aerobic exercise has been much touted in the past twenty years and for good cause. Every cell in your body requires a constant supply of oxygen, and, if you've been

---

If you're over thirty-five and your physical fitness is going to include anything more vigorous than brisk walking, then I suggest you have a doctor examine you and conduct a stress test to check for cardiovascular problems.

inactive for many years, many of them simply aren't getting their share. The more inactive you've been the better you're going to feel after a few months of exercise.

There are many stationary exercise machines on the market that will give you a good aerobic workout in the privacy of your own home. These include stationary bicycles (exercycles), stair-stepping exercisers, rowing machines, treadmills, and combinations. Thirty to forty minutes on one of these machines several days per week—enough to work up a sweat and breath a little hard for twenty minutes after a warm-up—will do wonders.

Those of you who are steadfastly committed to not getting too vigorous should fall back on walking or some other mildly aerobic exercise such as golfing, dancing, horseback riding, or even a regular game of ping pong. Remember to walk, not ride, the golf course.

Anaerobic Exercise

There are exercises—mostly strength-building exercises—that don't significantly increase oxygen consumption. Weight lifting and many forms of physical work fall into this anaerobic category. Though probably not as heart protective as aerobic exercise, many researchers now feel that strength training can also be supportive of general health.

Cautions

Unless you're very young and ambitious, don't do anything to exhaustion. If you take up some vigorous aerobic exercise, you needn't do it seven days a week; five should be more than enough. If you take up weight lifting, don't do it on two consecutive days. Your muscles need a rest. If you feel discomfort while exercising, especially dizziness or chest pain, stop instantly. It's time to visit your physician for a checkup.

If exercise becomes a pleasant habit, this chapter will have served you well. Remember, the secret of a good hundred-year survival plan is the combination of everything. All good things reinforce each other. Good food, good exercise, good vitamins, and good hormones, combined with a good attitude, spell victory.

CHAPTER THIRTEEN

Supplement for Life

THE LONG CONFLICT BETWEEN PROMOTERS OF VITAMIN AND mineral supplementation and their opponents has been pretty much won by the side that said vitamins could do you a lot of good. Oh, there are still a few die-hard oppositionists in the medical establishment, including Dr. David Kessler, head of the Food and Drug Administration. But when I tell you that polls show that four out of five doctors take vitamin E daily, I'm sure you'll agree that this particular health war is nearly over.

The reason it's ended the way it has is because there were just too many scientific studies published in the last twenty years showing that people who take vitamins suffer far less from the major debilitating illnesses—particularly heart disease and cancer—than people who don't. Take just one example—the study on vitamin C conducted by epidemiologists led by Dr. J. E. Enstrom at the University of California at Los Angeles and published in 1992. Their investigation was among the first fruits of a data base begun in 1971 when the National Center for Health Statistics began collecting extensive diet and nutrition information from 11,348 adults aged twenty-five to seventy-four. They began releasing their raw data in 1988 and Enstrom's group pounced. Reviewing the daily vitamin C intake of the participants, they divided them into three groups.

- Individuals with less than 50 mg daily.
- Individuals with 50 mg or more from food.
- Individuals with 50 mg or more from food, plus regular vitamin C supplementation, usually in the form of pills containing several hundred milligrams.

Would there be a relation between intake of C and mortality? You bet.

Men with the highest vitamin C intake—these were the participants who were taking supplementation—had a total number of deaths 35 percent lower than comparable groups in the total U.S. population. Their mortality due to cardiovascular diseases was 42 percent lower. Their cancer deaths were 22 percent lower. Women in the high-C group had lesser but still significant benefits: a 10 percent drop in total mortality, a 25 percent decline in heart disease deaths, and a 15 percent reduction in cancer deaths.

Such results were dramatically different from the people in the middle group who were getting 50 mg or more from their diets—in essence doing precisely what the official medical gurus have always recommended: eating a healthful diet but eschewing those worthless vitamins. How large was the life enhancing advantage of supplementation? Well, the group eating only a healthy diet showed only a 7 percent reduction in cardiovascular mortality for men as compared to the 42 percent in the supplemented group.

When my coauthor spoke to Dr. Enstrom several years ago, the UCLA epidemiologist noted that he had had a difficult time getting his study published because most of the major medical journals thought it too "controversial."

What a difference the last five years have made! Today only a terminally narrow-minded physician would discourage his patients from taking vitamin C, and most now recognize that multiple vitamins, too, are supplying us with insurance doses of nutrients we just might not be getting in sufficient quantities from the food we eat. There are many dozens of vitamins and minerals that your body is using daily to carry out chemical reactions, to manufacture hormones and enzymes, to maintain bones and nourish cells and keep you living at an optimal level instead of just crawling along. It is impossible to predict exactly what you'll need. Even the healthiest diet is likely to fall short in one area or another. Morevoer, as you get older your body is less efficient at extracting nutrients from the food you eat. Consequently, many older people are suffering from subtle indications of malnutrition.

Even the young and well nourished have every reason to supplement their diet, certainly in the area of the antioxidant vitamins and minerals. In our world, we need all the antioxidant protection we can get. Oh, I'm sure it's conceivable that a person living in a country with clean air and clean water, far from all sources of industrial and chemical pollution, and eating a perfect diet of natural, organically grown foods might not benefit all that much from additional supplementation. But there are so few humans left on this planet who live like that that we might have a hard time getting a sufficient number together to adequately test the hypothesis.

And not only do we face serious environmental health challenges—most of us daily—but we are also eating food grown on depleted farmland that no longer yields adequate quantities of essential nutrients, particularly trace elements. Much of what is now grown is deficient in selenium, for instance, which is absolutely essential to the production of glutathione peroxidase, one of your body's most potent internal antioxidants, and deficient in chromium, without which carbohydrates cannot be properly utilized for energy by your cells. Neither of these elements is necessary for the actual growth of plants, so the agricultural industry has no incentive to replace them in their depleted soil.

There are, of course, whole books written about the vitamins and minerals our bodies require. In the space of one chapter, I can't provide even a superficial examination of the more important ones. I simply want to convince you that supplementation is good for you. Doctors like myself, who have prescribed vitamins and minerals supplementally for decades, know that a significant proportion of our patients—and not necessarily very sick ones—show measurable improvements in health and energy when they go on a strong supplement program. It is no exaggeration at all to say that I have known hundreds of patients who scoffed at the idea of vitamin supplements and came back to see me a month later and scoffed no more. Nutritionally speaking, I run a subspeciality in making believers out of skeptics.

A SIMPLE VITAMIN PLAN

You will, of course, have your own sources for vitamins. Below, I simply recommend the total supplemental contents found in the six tablets I suggest that my patients take daily. I ask that they take two tablets at each meal because they're absorbed best then and because the digestive process itself triggers increased levels of free radical activity. Thus, they get protection with their food.

Vitamin A	10,000 IU
Beta carotene	15,000 IU
Vitamin D	100 IU
Vitamin C	1,200 mg
Vitamin B_1 (thiamine)	100 mg

Vitamin B_2 (riboflavin)	50 mg
Vitamin B_6 (pyridoxine)	25 mg
Vitamin B_{12}	100 mcg
Niacin	50 mg
Niacinamide	150 mg
Pantothenic acid	500 mg
Folic acid	800 mcg
Biotin	300 mcg
Choline	100 mg
Inositol	100 mg
Para-amino benzoic acid (PABA)	50 mg
Vitamin E (d-alpha tocopherol)	400 IU
Calcium	500 mg
Magnesium	500 mg
Potassium	99 mg
Iodine	150 mcg
Manganese (aspartate)	20 mg
Copper (gluconate)	2 mg
Boron (chelate)	1 mg
Zinc	20 mg
Molybdenum (chelate)	100 mcg
Chromium	200 mcg
Selenium	200 mcg
Vanadium (chelate)	25 mcg
Bioflavonoids (rutin, hesperidin)	100 mg

CHAPTER FOURTEEN

Choosing a Longevity Diet

You've all noticed the concern about diet—really a sort of mild national obsession—that's surfaced in the past two decades. Make sense? I'm afraid it does. If you plan to live a long and healthy life, you're simply going to have to think about the two or three pounds of food you put in your mouth each day. It can't help having a considerable effect on your health, since, over time, you are actually replacing the material substance of your present body with the molecular contribution provided by your daily diet.

Common sense is on the side of eating right. The only question is, what's right?

There are some general principles that apply to most of us, but the first point I want to emphasize is that good diet is highly individualized. Once we get past our "eat anything, feel great" teens and twenties, we should discover that the art of eating right is a process of self-testing. The food that's right for you is what keeps you looking trim, with healthy skin and hair; it's what makes you feel good day after day, full of energy, eager to go out and do things, not sluggish and sleepy and suffering from brain fog. It's food that you enjoy eating but that you don't find yourself obsessing over, like sugar addicts who are constantly dreaming of that next piece of pie or dish of ice cream.

Though we each have our own particular balance of fish and meat, vegetables and salads, potatoes, whole grains, pasta and rice that suits us, I don't doubt that you can benefit from a chapter's worth of basic dos and don'ts. Let's take a look.

WHAT HELPS; WHAT HURTS

I'm going to assume you plan to live to be a hundred and twenty. This is a challenging ambition, and, in spite of the genuinely remarkable pro-longevity hormones I've been telling you about, I don't think you're going to make it unless you use your food for two purposes.

First, of course, you want to build up your body with healthy nutrients. A powerful regimen of vitamins and minerals packaged in the best quality foods will maximize the functioning of all your metabolic systems. This will give you the strength to continue to grow and build new tissue, and will provide your body with a wide-ranging panoply of antioxidants—the molecular defense team that defuses free radicals as they're being formed in your body. Remember, as oxygen-breathing creatures, we are constantly creating damaging free radicals as the natural byproducts of just living. These molecular bad guys damage and kill our good cells and can open us right up to the main killers of the second half of life: atherosclerosis and cancer. So you're going to need the right foods (and nutritional supplements, too, as we discussed in the last chapter) to strengthen and protect you.

Secondly, it's going to be important for you not to misuse the pleasures of eating by blatantly eating the wrong things. There are foods—sugar, white flour, margarine, rancid oils—that simply aren't good for anyone anytime.

Take in a lot of those foods and you're tearing down the body that this book is dedicated to showing you how to build up. And then there are foods that are fine in moderation: meat, fish, fowl, eggs, butter. How much of these saturated fats you should be eating is very much a matter of individual metabolism. I don't think most people should be consuming huge quantities, but I'm not preaching a radically low-fat diet either. Some people seem to function well as carnivores; others do best with something fairly close to a vegetarian diet. I'm going to propose in this chapter an eating plan that seems to work well for the vast majority of my patients and which has plenty of scientific evidence to back it up. If you follow that plan and then modify it slightly in the direction of what makes you feel most energetic and healthy day in and day out, you should have no difficulty creating a truly formidable pro-longevity diet.

THE ANTI-FREE-RADICAL DIET

That's exactly what this chapter is going to introduce you to, for, as an ancient Chinese proverb puts it, "The beginning of wisdom is to call things by their right name."

The electron-hungry free radicals that I told you about in Chapter Seven are byproducts of just living. The reason that the animals on this planet—including humans— are capable of leading such incredibly active lives is because they use an incredible high activity fuel: oxygen. Watch the way a wood fire burns: it's consuming oxygen, as well as logs, for fuel. So do we consume oxygen in a more controlled fashion, and we pay the price. Our bodies have constructed a formidable network of defense against the almost explosively reactive substance that fuels it. Our bodies make every effort to stay saturated with antioxidants—substances that inhibit free radical formation and defuse the free radicals already formed. Nevertheless, it has been estimated that there are enough free radicals let loose in our bodies in every twenty-four-hour period to subject each and every one of our cells to a thousand hits by unbalanced electron-hunting molecules. This is war!

It turns out that many of the prime sources of pathologically active free radicals can be easily evaded via dietary manipulation. For example, we can avoid consuming processed unsaturated oils (particularly the more rancid ones) and stop eating highly processed foods stripped of essential protective anti-oxidants and other nutrients.

This is a decided departure from the outmoded "no eggs, less animal fat" dietary approach to minimizing the risk of cardiovascular disease.

The anti-free-radical diet establishes a five-pronged approach to combating free radicals.

- It reduces consumption of foods that metabolize readily into excess free radicals.
- It supplies optimal amounts of free radical scavenging nutrients.
- It provides ample quantities of those trace and ultra-trace nutrients necessary for normal metabolism—for healing, immunity, and manufacture of antioxidant enzymes.
- It utilizes nonoxidizing food preparation methods to minimize free radical lipid peroxidation before consumption.
- It reduces intake of fatty foods with high caloric density, leading to reduction of excess body fat, and reducing internal sources of lipid peroxide free radicals. (*Lipid* is a medical word meaning fat, and lipid peroxidation is a process whereby free radicals disrupt fatty membranes within and surrounding cells, a process, therefore, of cell destruction—just what you don't want your food to be doing to you. In the remainder of this chapter, I'll frequently be mentioning peroxidation as a bad quality caused by food you don't want to eat too much of.)

Unlike some rigidly restrictive nutritional regimens, the anti-free-radical diet doesn't take all the fun out of eating. You needn't swear off moderate amounts of properly prepared eggs, butter, shrimp, liver, and other foods high in dietary cholesterol that have long been mistakenly maligned as lethal.

This is not really a diet in the traditional sense, inasmuch as there are no meal plans to follow. What it is is an eating, cooking, and food-selection program designed to help you eat smarter, so that you receive the maximum possible protection from free-radical-induced illness.

Here are the pro-longevity guidelines that I and my patients live by.

***Reduce consumption of dietary fats and oils*—** especially the processed polyunsaturated or hydrogenated varieties—to 25 percent or less of total calories consumed.

Although essential fatty acids are necessary for healthy skin, arteries, blood, glands, nerves, and, indeed, all cells, most health experts agree on the wisdom of lowering total fat intake. They disagree, however, on how low is low enough. Some maintain no more than 10 percent—a truly Spartan requirement—of total calories is allowable. My recommendation is to stay in the more easily managed 20 to 25 percent range, paying careful to the sources, the processing and the quality of your fats and oils.

Moderating the amount of fat eaten is vital because dietary fats are the prime source of excess internal free radical production. Fats—especially polyunsaturated fats and oils—have a chemical composition that oxidizes readily, triggering chains of free radical reactions.

The untold part of the story is that reducing the quantity of fat is not nearly as crucial as eliminating the wrong kinds of fat. Contrary to popular mythology, it is not the saturated (animal) fats that are the "bad guys" and the polyunsaturated fats (liquid oils of vegetable or seed origin) that are the "good guys." It is exactly the reverse—especially if the oils have been exposed to light, heat, and air in the extraction, bottling, and food preparation process. And they almost always have been.

Saturated fats, such as we find in butter, eggs, beef, lamb, and pork, can be eaten more safely when prepared properly. The saturated fatty acids that they contain are not—under normal conditions—easily subject to the cell-damaging lipid peroxidation that I told you about a moment ago.

In sharp contrast, the polyunsaturated fats that are commercially processed (vegetable and seed oils) undergo extensive lipid peroxidation that damages their molecular structure. This begins the very moment these fats are extracted from the foods in which they naturally occur. Consumption of such chemically altered fats disrupts our normal metabolism, impairs cell membranes, and initiates the mutation process that contributes to plaque formation in the arteries, cancer, and arthritis. This is the reverse of pro-longevity with a vengeance. The richer the oil in polyunsaturated fatty acids and the longer it was exposed to heat, light, atmospheric oxygen, and trace amounts of metallic elements, the greater the health threat. The poorest quality oils are customarily used in the manufacture of salad dressings and mayonnaise, since their rancidity can be so easily masked by heavy seasoning.

Even the so-called cold-processed oils, premium priced in health food stores, cause damage to the arteries in excess. Just as soon as the oil is extracted from its source— the soybean, peanut, corn kernel, walnut, sesame seed, etc.—it begins to peroxidize.

Heating vegetable oils to fry foods greatly compounds the problem. When an oil is heated, the rate of peroxidation increases rapidly, doubling with every ten-degrees-centigrade rise in temperature.

Hydrogenation, such as takes place during the commercial preparation of margarine, vegetable shortenings, and products like nondairy creamers and nondairy whipped toppings, also converts polyunsaturated fats and oils into dangerous trans fatty acids. Most of the baked goods and junk food in your local supermarket are filled with hydrogenated oils, which have the commercially pleasing property of extending shelf life.

Do you protect your health by substituting margarine for butter? Hardly.

Margarine is clearly more toxic. Contrary to the image of the attractive Indian maiden on the package, by the time corn oil margarine reaches your table, it is completely unnatural. Not only have its original ingredients been drastically altered, but its free fatty acids have been combined with harsh chemicals and treated by petroleum-based solvents. The last defenders of this extraordinarily unattractive food began to lose their confidence in 1993 when Dr. Walter Willett and his team of researchers published the latest chapter in the findings of the Harvard Nurses Study, a many-decades-long project following the health fortunes of 85,000 nurses. It turned out that the women who were eating the equivalent of four or more teaspoons of margarine daily had a 66 percent greater risk of developing heart disease than women whose consumption was very low or who didn't consume the synthetic butter at all. As for butter itself, there was no indication of increased cardiovascular risk among the women who ate it.

Here are some suggestions that will help you reduce dietary fats and maximize both the length and the quality of your life.

When eating beef, lamb, pork, or veal, always select the freshest, leanest meat available. Aged meats owe their enhanced flavor to rancidity. Trim all visible fat before preparation. To satisfy your beef hunger, choose dishes such as casseroles or stews that provide smaller individual portions of meat than a roast or a steak. When a recipe calls for hamburger, buy the leanest variety, precook it, and drain off all the fat before adding it to the dish.

Frequently substitute fish and lean fowl for other meat. Even the leanest beef you can buy has more than twice as much total fat as skinless white meat from chicken, fish, or turkey. Remove as much of the skin and subcutaneous fat as possible before cooking or eating poultry.

Eliminate fried foods from your diet. Learn to become adept at greaseless cooking. Use greaseless, nonstick cookware (Teflon is one popular, easily available brand), which never needs oils or fats to keep food from sticking to pots or pans. Slow-roast meats, fish, and fowl.

Use dairy products with the lowest fat content, such as 1 percent fat cottage cheese or nonfat skim milk. Cottage cheese and milk labeled as containing 1 percent fat by weight actually contain 10 percent of total calories as fat.

Whole milk contains 40 percent of calories as butter fat and cholesterol. Heating and stirring the milk during pasteurization speeds peroxidation of fatty acids and cholesterol, contributing to free radical disease.

Be wary of imitation dairy products. Pseudo-sour cream, for example, is often made with hydrogenated oils and has no place on an anti-free-radical diet. But nonfat cream cheese, yogurt, and sour cream are now easily available.

Substitute vinegar, lemon juice, garlic, onion, or herbs for salad oils and dressings, tomato and other fruit juices for rich sauces and gravies. Garlic and onion have the additional benefit of being rich sources of dietary anti-oxidants.

Limit your intake of hidden fats. Restrict your consumption of pies, cakes, puddings, ice cream, and similar desserts. Non-fat ice cream is now available, but it remains high in sugar.

Avoid the "white plague" foods—white flour, white rice, refined white sugar.

Much of the American public now suffers from a form of "over-consumption malnutrition." Their diet contains too many calories that have been stripped by the food industry of most of the trace nutrients necessary for protection from external and internal pollution. The high-speed milling of grains such as wheat, rice, and corn results in the reduction or removal of more than twenty nutrients, including essential fatty acids and the majority of minerals and essential trace elements. Ideally, your refined carbohydrate intake should be close to zero—no breads, crackers, cereals, pastas, or snacks made from highly processed, nutrient-depleted starches. If the food says "enriched," be especially cautious.

In comparision with the nutrients that naturally exist in wheat grain as it's growing in the field, the approximate percentage of each removed in the production of white bread is as follows:

90 percent of the vitamin A,
77 percent of the vitamin B_1,
80 percent of the vitamin B_2,
81 percent of vitamin B_3,
72 percent of vitamin B_6,
77 percent of vitamin B_{12},
50 percent of the pantothenic acid,

86 percent of the vitamin E,
67 percent of the folic acid,
60 percent of the calcium,
40 percent of the chromium,
89 percent of the cobalt,
76 percent of the iron,
85 percent of the magnesium,
86 percent of the manganese,
71 percent of the phosphorus,
77 percent of the potassium,
16 percent of the selenium,
30 percent of the choline,
and 78 percent of the zinc and copper!

At most, only four of these vitamins—B_1, B_2, B_3, and iron—are put back in the so-called enrichment process. And—if a deficiency does not exist—iron supplementation has the potential to accelerate free radical damage in your body.

Refined white sugar likewise lacks most vital nutrients, including the ingredients, such as chromium, needed for its own metabolism. Thus each spoonful you consume (the average American's annual intake of sugar and high fructose corn syrup is up to 137 pounds) steals the nutrients needed to digest it from other foods in the diet or from reserves in the body. Insulin cannot metabolize sugar in the abssence of adequate chromium.

Many of the enzymes involved in free radical protection—your body's own internally produced antioxidant team—including catalase, superoxide dismutase, and glutathione peroxidase—require the very nutrients lost in the refining process. Without these control enzymes, free radicals are generated at an ever-increasing rate.

Other molecules that neutralize unwanted free radicals include beta carotene, vitamin E, vitamin C, the trace element selenium, zinc, copper, manganese, and the amino acid cysteine. Without these substances—all virtually zapped out of natural foods during processing—the body cannot protect itself.

The best way to cut down on your consumption of unrefined carbohydrates is to up your intake of natural, unrefined foods, particularly whole grain products and green and yellow vegetables, which should ideally make up about 60 to 65 percent of your total daily calories. Here are some tips for an unrefined, healthy diet.

Read labels carefully. Choose sugar-free whole grain cereals and whole grain breads. Eat brown rice and whole wheat buckwheat, or soy pasta products. Steer clear of products with the telltale "enriched" notation. When you translate enriched into honest English, what you get is "almost totally impoverished."

Cook from scratch. There are hidden sugars in hundreds of processed foods we don't normally think of as sweet—canned vegetables, salad dressings, catsup, biscuit mix, TV dinners, mayonnaise, steak sauce. Hydrogenated fats and oils are commonly found in factory-made, processed foods.

Avoid foods that contain disguised refined sugars. These include sucrose, dextrose, corn sweeteners, corn syrup, maltose, invert sugar, raw sugar, brown sugar, turbinade, fructose. Most so-called raw and brown sugar is just refined white sugar colored with a little molasses.

Be wary of sugar-free soft drinks or so-called diet drinks, especially those that are cola-flavored. They contain excessive phosphates, which disrupt normal calcium metabolism. And evidence is accumulating to incriminate aspartame in many adverse affects on the body.

Eat mainly whole foods—fresh fruits and vegetables, whole grains, peas, and beans—whenever possible. Eat the food whole (the fruit instead of the juice) and the entire vegetable (potatoes with skins). Train yourself to shop mainly around the fringes of your supermarket, the outer aisles where the fresh produce, dairy products, meat and fish are sold. Avoid the inner aisles where the brightly colored packages of highly processed foods are kept.

Increase dietary fiber—dietary fiber binds bile acids and promotes their speedier movement through the digestive tract, thus reducing the time they're subjected to putrefaction, oxidation, and reabsorption.

Increasing your consumption of dietary fiber is easily accomplished.

1. *Eat more root vegetables* such as potatoes, parsnips, cabbage, yams, etc. Other high-fiber vegetables are spinach, beets, Brussels sprouts, carrots, cauliflower, turnips, broccoli, and eggplant.
2. *Eat whole-grain bread*, preferably four slices a day. There is very little fiber value to breads made of milled white flour.
3. *Start every day with a high-fiber breakfast cereal* (oatmeal, whole-grain or rolled wheat, millet, buckwheat, corn and barley grits). Be wary of the ready-to-eat varieties, which are generally low in fiber.
4. *Add miller's bran or oat bran to your favorite recipes.* It has an innocuous texture and flavor. Be adventurous. Sprinkle bran on a salad, add it to your home-baked bread, stir it into a main dish casserole. But, good as it is, bran contains only one constituent of dietary fiber and is no substitute for a complete variety of whole-grain foods.

Reduce salt consumption—no matter how often you've heard it, it bears repeating: Cut back on salt. Not simply because of the link between excessive sodium intake and high blood pressure, but also because cell walls damaged by free radicals lose some of their ability to maintain a proper sodium gradient. Excessive sodium leaks into a cell that is already compromised, causing further metabolic impairment. Small blood capillaries, damaged by free radicals, leak plasma into soft tissues, causing swelling and edema. A free-radical-damaged sodium pump is less able to remove excess sodium from within cells.

Lowering your salt intake is easier said than done. Food processors add it to foods that rarely taste salty. For example, would you suspect it to be an ingredient in Kellogg's corn flakes? Jell-O chocolate pudding? Low-fat cottage cheese? All three have salt added, but the real surprise is how much. One serving of pudding contains 404 mg of sodium chloride—one third the amount in a steeped-in-brine dill pickle.

Since salt is a likely ingredient in any processed food not specifically labeled "No salt added," here are the most practical ways to cut back.

1. *Reduce voluntary salting.* Do not use a salt shaker at the table. When cooking, substitute garlic, onion powder, kelp powder, herbs, and natural spices in recipes that specify salt.
2. *Limit your use of high-salt condiments*—soy sauce, for example, and prepared steak sauces, gravies, and relishes.
3. *Restrict your intake of salt-laden foods*, including smoked fishes, delicatessen-style meats, canned soups, pickles, pretzels, potato chips, and similar snacks.

Learn to cook the anti-free-radical way—More often than you might realize, it's not *what* you cook but how you cook that causes health problems. As a general rule, the faster the food is cooked and the higher the heat levels that it's exposed to, the more health-destructive the changes that occur. Heat speeds up the chemical reactions of peroxidation.

Here are four rules for anti-free-radical cooking:

1. *Limit broiling over hot coals.* If you're one of millions of suburban homeowners who relish backyard patio cooking, you won't welcome this news: Your cherished charcoal broiler is a dangerous free radical generator. Charring food oxidizes it, producing free radical precursors, and this is the reason that charbroiled foods are carcinogenic. That sizzling steak (hamburger, hot dog, chicken breast), salted, seasoned, and grilled to tasty perfection, becomes coated with compounds—similar to those found in tobacco tars—called aromatic polynuclear hydrocarbons. They generate massive doses of free radicals, including singlet oxygen against which the body has little inherent defense. In fact, the smoke from a single steak's fat drippings contains as much of the carcinogen benzopyrene as the smoke from approximately three cartons of cigarettes—i.e., six hundred coffin nails.

   Grilled hamburger presents a special problem. Because of its high fat content and the large surface area exposed to air and heat, it is the most easily oxidized of all meats. In addition, iron and copper (potent free radical catalysts) are crushed out of the meat's cells and into the fat during the grinding process, accelerating its oxidation, making it particularly dangerous, especially if the beef is a few days old.

   The solution is to buy your hamburger fresh ground and extra lean and use it at once. Better yet, grind your own meat. Steer clear of fast-food burgers. And, if you can't give up your backyard grill, trim all visible fat from steaks, chops, and ribs, and take both skin and fat off the chicken.

2. *Rarely or never fry foods.* The oxidation of the fat used in frying added to the oxidation of the fat found in the food itself add up to a double whammy. Even animal fats—chicken, pork chops, fish, or eggs—normally thought of as saturated, do contain unsaturated fatty acids and cholesterol, both of which oxidize easily.

Animal experiments have shown oxidized cholesterol
to be so damaging that if as little as one percent of
the cholesterol in your diet is consumed in its oxidized
form, atherosclerosis may result.

Here's what that means in practical terms.

Eggs are okay in moderation unless you fry them.
In its natural state or when a fresh egg is either soft-
boiled or poached with intact yolk unexposed to air, its
cholesterol content remains unoxidized and is an excellent
free radical scavenger. The situation is reversed when
the egg is fried, scrambled, or cooked into a recipe. Then
the cholesterol is partially oxidized into a number of cell-
damaging, toxic by-products. The same holds true for all
animal protein foods containing preformed cholesterol,
including most meats and many types of shellfish, poultry,
and seafood. Fresh baked, poached, or steamed, with all
visible fat removed, these are high quality foods; fried
they become toxic.

Be doubly wary of restaurant fried foods, where
highly oxidized (rancid) fat is often used over and over
again.

3. *Learn to cook without overcooking.* Easy advice to follow.
   Invest in a crock pot and/or a wok. Both methods rarely
   allow foods to exceed 212 degrees, the boiling point of
   water—below that, lipid peroxidation takes place more
   slowly. When using a wok, always add some water (or a
   minimum of oil) to prevent food from getting too hot.

4. *Avoid using aluminum cookware.* Ordinarily, aluminum
   cookware would not be a problem because the human
   body does not absorb much aluminum. However, studies
   indicate that aluminum does build up in the tissues of
   some disease victims. Aluminum deposition has been
   proven to occur in the arteries of atherosclerosis patients,
   and in the brains of Alzheimer's victims and some types of
   Parkinson's sufferers. Therefore, it probably makes sense
   to limit your exposure as much as possible, especially
   since aluminum is already widely used as a food additive
   and is in our drinking water and our medicines.

Eat an abundance of fresh whole grains and vegeta-bles—and do so as soon as possible after purchase.

While all methods of food storage result in critical nutrient loss, some are decidedly worse than others. Freezing food delays deterioration, but major nutrient losses can occur if the food is blanched prior to quick freezing. Prolonged storage will produce vitamin loss and progressive lipid peroxidation.

For instance, asparagus left unrefrigerated for three days prior to use has lost most of its B-complex vitamins before you ever get it home. The same holds true, in varying degrees, for other veggies. Ideally you should buy fresh-picked produce at farm stores and markets and only as much as you can serve and eat shortly after purchase.

Eat an abundance of foods rich in vitamin C, beta carotene, vitamin E, the B-complex vitamins, and the trace elements selenium, manganese, potassium, and zinc so that you will help your body produce the dozen or more antioxidant control systems that regulate free radical reactions.

I place such emphasis on fresh, whole foods in their natural state, because these nutrients must be present in sufficient quantity and in proper ratio to each other to activate free radical defenses.

You can get the highest concentration of vitamin C from green peppers, broccoli, Brussels sprouts, strawberries, spinach, oranges, cabbage, grapefruit, and cauliflower. To beef up the beta carotene content of your diet, select lots of carrots, sweet potatoes, cantaloupe, apricots, peaches, cherries, tomatoes, and asparagus. The fruits and vegetables richest in the B-complex vitamins are peas, corn, potatoes, lima beans, and artichokes.

Here are some general rules that apply to choosing and eating fresh foods.

1. *When shopping for food, give top priority to freshness.* Of the alternatives, frozen should be second choice, provided you can be certain the produce has not been blanched or thawed and refrozen. Third place goes to dried foods. They deteriorate quite slowly, but lose most vitamin C and vitamin A content because of the high heat involved in the drying process. In last place, canned foods. Canning of fruits and vegetables causes the most nutrient loss—as much as 50 percent of such potent antioxidants as vitamn C and the B-complex vitamins.

2. *Eat your vegetables raw whenever possible.* Concoct your own nonfat salad dressings by combining whatever spices, herbs, and condiments you like with nonfat yogurt, nonfat buttermilk, or 1 percent low-fat cottage cheese. Most modern cookbooks have a variety of recipes for delicious oil-free salad dressings. When you must cook vegetables, undercook them. They should retain some crispness. Steaming is less damaging than boiling.

3. *Arrange to eat fresh foods within three days of purchase.* Return frozen foods that reveal telltale refrozen signs when opened (food covered with ice crystals or a sheet of ice). Keep close track of food stored in your freezer. Check "use by" dates on containers (yes, they're often there, but you have to hunt for them).

Avoid excess caffeine, soda, and alcohol—as well as chlorinated drinking water containing chemicals.

Simply put, people fare better without excess caffeine. Drinking more than five cups of coffee a day considerably increases your risk of arterial disease and associated ailments.

Soft drinks, especially cola-flavored varieties (sugar-free or not) skew the body's delicate calcium/phosphorus balance, already a problem since the typical American diet contains twice as much phosphorus as calcium instead of the optimal one-to-one ratio.

Where does all the extra phosphorus come from? Red meats have many times more phosphorus than calcium, another good reason to rely more on poultry and fish for high-quality protein. Many carbonated beverages have phosphate buffers to prevent the carbon dioxide from forming carbonic acid. Thirdly, extra phosphorus comes from processed foods laced with preservatives, many of which are phosphate-based.

Why is the calcium/phosphorus ratio so important? When it is out of balance, excessive calcium tends to leak into cells, deposit in soft tissues, and accelerate aging. When cells are overwhelmed by calcium, they die.

One or two moderate-sized alcoholic beverages a day—no more—is a safe limit for most persons, except for pregnant women, people with seriously compromised health, and those with a predisposition for alcoholism. Alcohol metabolizes to become acetaldehyde, a potent free radical precursor and cross-linker.

Water is no less important to our bodies than food, yet we have good reason to fear for the quality and safety of our water supply. Public water supplies often contain numerous added chemicals that are possibly harmful. Artificially softened water can also be dangerous because of its excess salt and its occasional abundance of lead and cadmium, two of the more potent toxins.

I advise that you drink well water only when you are certain the well is far away from any source of commercial toxic waste and that, if you are suspicious of your local supply, you have it tested. Otherwise drink bottled spring or distilled water or equip your tap with a tested and effective water purifier. Reverse osmosis water purifiers are quite good, especially in conjunction with activated charcoal.

When planning meals to suit the anti-free-radical diet, here are the foods I recommend you eat each day:

Vegetables. At least two generous servings of a variety of fresh vegetables, especially those known to be the chief food sources of the important antioxidants beta carotene, vitamin C, and vitamin B complex. That list includes: artichokes, asparagus, beet greens, snap beans, lima beans, navy beans, broccoli, Brussels sprouts, cabbage, carrots, cauliflower, collards, chard, yellow corn, kale, kohlrabi, lentil, mushrooms, green peas, pumpkin, sauerkraut, snow pea pods, spinach, squash, succotash, winter squash, sweet potatoes, tomatoes, turnip greens, turnips, water chestnuts, and zucchini.

Salads. Two servings a day from any combination of raw vegetables. You can add extra anti-free-radical potency by the liberal use of chicory, Chinese cabbage, cucumber, endives, escarole, lettuce, parsley, pimento, chives, red and green peppers, dandelion greens, watercress, radishes, scallions, garlic, onions, and leeks. Season salads with lemon juice, herbs, or oil-free dressings. Olive oil on salads is least likely to be peroxidized because it is a monounsaturate.

Fruits. Two to three fresh servings a day, not canned, cooked or juiced, with the selection depending on individual taste and what is seasonally available. Chief fruit sources of antioxidant nutrients are apricots, bananas, cantaloupe, all melons, oranges, tangerines, papayas, peaches, plums, prunes, lemons, limes, pineapples, tomatoes, black currants, raspberries, rhubarb, and strawberries.

Protein Foods. Two servings a day consisting of the following: four- to six-ounce portions of lean beef, pork, veal, or lamb, no more than two to three times a week. As often as possible, replace red meat with chicken, turkey, or fish. Use only water-packed canned tuna.

Eggs. One or two a day, up to ten a week, preferably fresh-boiled or poached, with yolks intact, not scrambled, fried, or cooked into other dishes.

Cereals and breadstuffs. Two to six servings a day of unrefined whole-grain products. These include such breakfast cereals as oatmeal, all bran, and shredded wheat, pasta, breads, muffins, or crackers made from whole grain flours, and brown rice. Breads sparingly spread with butter, never margarine.

Dairy products. Drink only nonfat skim milk. Use nonfat cheeses and other dairy products.

Beverages. Decaffeinated coffee is fine (no more than three cups a day of nondecaffeinated coffee); milk—no more than three cups of nonfat skim milk per day; alchoholic beverages—limited to a maximum of 2 ounces of liquor, 8 ounces of wine, or two 12-ounce cans of beer; avoid most soft drinks. There is no limit on naturally carbonated spring water.

Desserts and snacks. Choose fresh fruit, dried fruit, puddings, sherbets, and gelatins made at home from sugar-free recipes. For an occasional treat, have a handful of freshly cracked, unsalted nuts; fresh-roasted chestnuts; dried raisins; or a slice of fat-free, homemade sponge or angel food cake.

Eating the anti-free-radical way is not difficult and can easily be made very pleasurable. Learn to shop, cook, and eat so that your food intake prepares you for a hardy old age. It can be an exciting adventure, for you have much to gain—a longer, healthier, happier life.

CHAPTER FIFTEEN

A Lifetime Plan for Hormones

WHAT SHOULD YOUR HORMONE PLAN BE? WILL IT BE BOLD AND costly? Conservative and limited? Nonexistent? Nothing in this book is meant to suggest you simply *must* take hormones. You may want to wait a few years and see how things develop. I wouldn't blame you. If your health is excellent and your energy where you want it to be, you can afford to wait.

Nonetheless, it would be feeble and disingenuous of me to pretend, after all that we've written, that I doubt the benefits of hormone replacement. I've treated too many people, read too many medical papers, and talked to too many other doctors to believe that the effects of the pro-longevity hormones are anything less than extraordinary.

Though we cannot say for certain what the results of long-term use of HGH, DHEA, melatonin, and the sex hormones will be, the evidence we now possess makes it reasonable to surmise that the vast majority of people who receive them will feel better, behave more vigorously, look younger, and live longer than those around them who do not. The evidence for long-term administration of pro-longevity hormones, other than the sex hormones, has not been accu-

mulated in mass, but is not by any means totally lacking. I
know of a small number of senior citizens who have been
taking HGH for more than a decade without untoward side
effects and to their complete satisfaction. There are many
people who have been taking DHEA even longer. We also
have the records of tens of thousands of children and
adolescents who have taken HGH for periods as long as
ten years.

It seems that we can say that if there are any unexpected long-term side effects to the pro-longevity hormones, the vast majority of people escape them, certainly
in the first ten years of use.

How does one decide—really decide—on use? Should
you change the hand that nature has dealt you, replace the
threes and fours with queens, kings, and aces? Frankly all
I can think to say is: How can you ask? Do we choose sick-
ness when we're offered health, choose prison in place of
freedom, chains instead of wings, death instead of life? If
we have failed in this book to convince you of the merits of
the pro-longevity hormones, then, indeed, we have signally
failed.

As I said before, all life is a taking of risks. Are the risks
involved in hormone replacement—and it would be unfair
to suggest there are none—worth the taking? Well, there's
one thing I know about you, you're getting older. You may be
in middle age or approaching it. You may be on the edge of
old age or already firmly there. Wherever you are, you can
make a difference in your life right now. The older you are,
the more crucial these decisions will be. But the decision is
there, present, I think, for everyone who's past youth.

No question that I'm proposing a radical rearrange-
ment of life. Old age, step back. We may soon have to
invent a new term for some of those years. There's now
abundant evidence that for many of us, our sixties, seventies, and eighties will not be old age but simply a pleasant
prolongation of our middle years. That is the real potential

of the pro-longevity hormones. What if middle age were to extend from forty to ninety? It will. For millions and eventually tens of millions of men and women, this is how life is going to be. Old age postponed—not by years but by decades. And, when it comes, the havoc, debilitation, and destruction that it brings—and, why be coy, this is exactly what old age does bring for most folks eventually—will be sensibly and measurably lessened.

In the last chapter of this book, we are going to speculate on the ultimate prolongation of life—stretching the human lifespan beyond its present limit of a hundred and twenty years. That will be a short but interesting survey of the latest approaches. But that will be pure speculation.

What we now have before us—not speculative at all but very, very real—is a solidly based prospect of living in good mental and physical health past a hundred. That is what the hormone breakthrough has done for us, and I personally find the prospect totally exilarating. That's why I take these hormones myself. What I'm going to do in the next few pages is briefly summarize the benefits that you can expect from hormones as we've described them in the book so far. Then I'll outline, as best I can without ever having met you, a bare-bones personal hormone plan. From it—with the help of your physician—you should be able to create your own individualized hormone replacement plan.

WHY TAKE HORMONES?

Look again at the basic areas that pro-longevity hormones reinforce, strengthen, and protect. Age brings decline. For each of us at a different rate and in different areas or aspects of the body. Even at forty, we may not sleep as well or have the boundless energy of a college student. So different parts of the following outline will be of greater or lesser interest to each one of you. Certainly there are categories—simple physical strength, for instance—that all of us lose as we get older and that all of us must seek to protect or regain.

But more significant than that is something I fear we haven't emphasized sufficiently in this book because our attention has been so concentrated on explaining the particular merits of each hormone. That's the merit of all of them together, the way nature gave them to us. I'm sure you remember in Chapter Two our description of the whole interrelated lineup of endocrine hormones. They do work in harmony together. They are a harmony, a metabolic music without which you would literally come unstrung. What you need if you're to hold on to a portion of the irreplaceable vitality of youth is not any one of the anti-aging hormones, but a combination of all of them.

Before we look at that combination, let's briefly glance at the benefit column for the pro-longevity hormones.

TEN HORMONAL ENHANCEMENTS

Physical Strength. Nothing ambiguous here. Youthful levels of human growth hormone are critical to maintaining muscular strength. Testosterone as well, the most powerful anabolic steroid in the human body is essential for both men and women, although in widely differing ratios, and estrogen, since it supports a woman's physical strength at any age, will definitely have a significant effect on strength maintenance postmenopausally.

Energy. HGH indirectly potentiates energy by increasing muscle mass and decreasing fat. An increase in energy is one of the most commonly observed effects of DHEA. And almost any woman who replaces estrogen or any man who replaces testosterone will tell you that they can go further, faster with replacement doses of these essential hormones than they can without them. Thyroid hormone (see Appendix One) will definitely have a powerful positive effect on the 10 to 20 percent of older people whose thyroid levels become low.

Immune System Function. There is powerful evidence from both human and animal studies to show that HGH and DHEA can restore immune system functions that have been weakened by age. And animal studies seem to show that both HGH and melatonin (and perhaps DHEA) help to regenerate the thymus gland, one of the main motors of our immune system. Such benefits are one of the main reasons for calling these substances pro-longevity hormones.

Maintaining Life Enthusiasm; Countering Depression. It has been my experience that few things more quickly revive enthusiasm for living than replacement doses of the hormones we had when we were young. Depression often vanishes in the face of HGH, DHEA, or the sex hormones, although in cases of severe clinical depression, the problem is more complex and requires a psychiatrist's guidance.

Mental Sharpness; Memory. People's brains work better when their levels of hormones are what they were when young. It's as simple and exciting as that. As one doctor well-versed in testosterone administration put it to me, "Old guys get their brains back." The hormones work for old girls, too. HGH and DHEA also have documented effects on memory and mental function.

Healthy Bones. HGH produces small but significant increases in bone density and strength. And the contribution of the sex hormones to the treatment and prevention of osteoporosis is well known.

Sex Function. Without proper levels of the sex hormones, sex is limited or nonexistent. With youthful levels, sex can be exciting far into old age. The choice is yours.

Sleep. In the last few years, melatonin has become legendary for its sleep-inducing properties. But don't forget that for many people DHEA improves sleep significantly.

Skin Quality; Appearance. Although most of the anti-aging hormones improve skin quality, the hands-down champs are estrogen in post-menopausal women and HGH in older folks whose skin is becoming thin. I've seen the parchment-like skin on the back of the hands of an eighty-seven year old man begin to thicken in as little as two months after replacement doses of HGH begin to be administered.

Longevity. I think the basic conclusion is clear: The pro-longevity hormones will increase length of life—we just don't know yet by how much.

THE LIFETIME PRO-LONGEVITY HORMONE TREATMENT PLAN

Now for recommendations. Let me state once again, for the record, that hormones are not to be taken lightly and that I believe you would be very foolish to undertake hormone replacement on your own, even if you could devise a method of procuring these largely prescription items. The first thing you should be doing is finding yourself an experienced and open-minded physician. If you find such an individual and there are some of the pro-longevity hormones he (or she) hasn't worked with, I encourage you to take on the task of going to a medical library and photo-copying some of the articles referenced at the end of this book. After all, if you're actually going to extend your life by a couple of decades, you can probably afford to spend a couple of hours making things easy for your overworked personal physician.

Here is what I recommend.

Men through the Decades

AGE FORTY TO FIFTY:

- *Melatonin*—a small bedtime dose—usually 3 mg but perhaps as little as 0.1 mg if drowsiness occurs the next day—is advisable in these years. The dose should be adjusted to your comfort. No lab tests are necessary.

- *DHEA*—is appropriate now. Ask your doctor to have levels of DHEAS in your blood drawn and measured. If you are below 2500 ng/ml, then supplementation may be advisable. I usually recommend 25 to 50 mg per day, but some men take 100 mg or more without any side effects.

AGE FIFTY TO SIXTY:

- *Testosterone*—this is a good time to measure your levels. If you come in at less than 400 ng/dl, talk to your physician about possible testosterone replacement. First, however, he should examine your prostate and do a PSA test to ensure that your prostate gland shows no indications of cancer. That would be a definite contra-indication for testosterone treatment. If the tests are satisfactory, your doctor will work out a treatment plan that gets your testosterone level close to 800 ng/dl. It may require the averaging of several blood tests over a period of some weeks to determine if you are receiving an appropriate dose.

- *Human Growth Hormone*—I tell those of my patients who are interested in a hormonal approach and who can afford it that this may be the best time to begin—before really serious depletion of HGH affects their general health. I know of no sixty-year-olds who are as physically strong as they were at forty, much less twenty. Ask your physician to get a baseline measurement of your somatomedin-C levels, and unless your level is unusually high for your age (over 300 ng/ml), consider therapy. Four units weekly is a reasonable dose. I would not recommend that you go higher than six to eight units weekly unless your physician can give you very sound reasons for such a step. You will recall that at higher doses side effects are more common.

- *Melatonin*—you may wish to consider raising your bedtime dose of melatonin. Most men who sleep well have no reason to go higher than 3 mg daily.

- *DHEA*—you may wish to increase your dose up to a maximum of 100 mg.

AGE SIXTY TO A HUNDRED AND TEN:

- Your physician should be measuring your blood levels of DHEA, somatomedin-C, and testosterone yearly to keep them within a normal, healthy range. If you are taking testosterone, have your prostate and your PSA levels checked yearly or even twice yearly. In this age bracket, 500 ng/dl is quite a healthy and sufficient level for testosterone. Increase melatonin if sleep problems occur.

Women through the Decades

AGE FORTY TO FIFTY:

- *Melatonin*—as for men, a small bedtime dose of melatonin—usually 3 mg, but perhaps as little as 0.1 mg if drowsiness occurs the next day—is advisable. The dose should be adjusted to comfort. No lab tests are necessary.

- *DHEA*—have your levels of DHEAS drawn and measured, and, if you're below 2500 ng/ml, you may want to supplement with 25 mg daily.

- *Hormone Replacement Therapy*—since the first indications of menopause will probably begin in this decade, as your periods grow more infrequent, you should consider hormonal replacement. Capsules containing tri-estrogen combined with natural progesterone taken twice daily is, in my opinion, the best approach. Talk to your physician about having your blood levels of testosterone measured and, if they're low, small quantities of testosterone (in conjunction with estrogen) may be desirable.

AGE FIFTY TO SIXTY:

- *Human Growth Hormone*—for women, as for men, this may be the time to begin. A desirable dose is usually in the area of 4 units weekly.

- *DHEA*—continue checking your levels of DHEAS. Many women who didn't begin in their forties will begin taking DHEA in this decade.

- *Hormone Replacement Therapy*—you will definitely have arrived at menopause in this decade. The same approach to hormone replacement that I described for women in their forties applies to you.

- *Melantonin*—consider raising your dose if sleep problems occur. Three mg daily at bedtime is the usual dose, but more is safe if needed to achieve restful sleep.

AGE SIXTY TO A HUNDRED AND TEN:

- Your need for HGH, DHEA, and possibly melatonin will continue, and your doses and levels should be monitored and maintained. Your replacement doses of estrogen, progesterone, and perhaps testosterone will be fine-tuned as you grow older. Increase bedtime doses of melatonin if sleep problems occur.

YOU'RE ON YOUR WAY

Let me utter the obvious just one more time. The pro-longevity hormones are providing you with the hormonal levels that gave you the vitality of youth. But their effects—remarkable as they are—will only be fully appreciated by men and women who have made a total commitment to health. Smoking, drinking, drug abuse, and similar destructive habits can wreck the health of a twenty-five-year-old, so have no doubt that they can certainly destroy you as you grow older. Good hormone levels can't even begin to compensate for self-destruction.

I think you now have the ability to formulate a comprehensive plan for self-preservation, one that will give you a better than equal chance of passing a hundred and aiming for the record books. More important, I think you can do that standing on your own two legs and enjoying every day of your life. But the exact details of your plan must be put together by you and followed with a fair degree of discipline. If you do that, then your prospects of a long and healthy life will be immeasurably strengthened.

I certainly hope that each and every one of my readers will choose to do exactly that.

Now let's turn to the last chapter and see what the wizards of longevity are planning for the future. If some of their schemes come to fruition, then by the time you reach a hundred, we may have written a new book telling you how to live to a hundred-and-fifty. It's not impossible, you know.

Administering the Hormones

THE BEST TIME OF DAY

Most of the pro-longevity hormones seem to work better when taken at a particular time of day. My recommendations are as follows:

Human Growth Hormone—take in the evening within a few hours of bedtime to mimic the body's own cycle.

DHEA—take within an hour or two of rising.

Melatonin—take at night, usually within a half hour before you plan to sleep.

Estrogen and progesterone—take twice during the day at a twelve-hour interval.

Testosterone—if you are using a cream or gel, apply in the evening an hour or two before bedtime to mimic the body's own production. If you are taking an injection, this will be administered weekly or biweekly, and the time of day is not significant. The same obviously applies to a pellet implanted twice yearly.

THE BEST FORM IN WHICH TO TAKE THEM

- Human Growth Hormone is always taken by injection, usually four times weekly.
- DHEA can be taken in a tablet, in a powder-filled capsule, or in a capsule containing micronized powder suspended in oil.
- Melatonin is taken in capsules, tablets, or in a sublingual tablet that dissolves under the tongue.
- Estrogen and progesterone are best taken together in a capsule containing the micronized hormones suspended in oil. There is no reason for the pharmacist to be separating the hormones into two capsules and charging you more. If you have had a hysterectomy, you will not need progesterone. In that case, however, it will be more desirable for you to take a small dose of testosterone to help protect your bone.
- Testosterone is usually applied as a cream or gel or imbedded in a patch. It can also be injected (in my opinion, the most effective approach), but many people find the injection psychologically distressing because the needle is quite large. Or it can be implanted in the buttock in a pellet twice yearly.

CHAPTER SIXTEEN

The Future of Anti-Aging

HORMONES ARE AN IMPORTANT PIECE OF THE LONGEVITY PUZZLE, and this book has been a progress report on their use and development. We now know we will change and extend life significantly through the use of pro-longevity hormones. What of the other pieces—the non-hormonal keys to extended life?

There are many possibilities currently being investigated. One of the most promising and complicated involves altering and improving our gene pool.

Scientists are well aware that some genes improve our likelihood of long-term survival and others directly hinder us. One particular gene—the apo-E gene—has received extended scrutiny in the past few years. This gene not only produces a substance essential for transporting cholesterol in the bloodstream but, in the wrong form, predisposes people to Alzheimer's disease by mechanisms yet unknown. People can have three different types of the apo-E gene, and it turns out that only one of these is consistently found in individuals who survive past a hundred years. The other two forms are much more common in people who die at younger ages of heart disease—and one form of the gene is extremely prevalent in Alzheimer's patients, especially those who are stricken with this brain-killing disease early in life. If we can alter these genes, it will be possible to extend life for many people and to greatly decrease the incidence of a dreadful disease.

Doctors now know that it will soon be theoretically possible to correct bad genes or add good ones. They've already done it with lower life forms. Experiments on *Drosophila melanogaster*—the common fruit fly—have given the tiny creature extra copies of a gene that signals its cells to produce protective antioxidants. Fruit fly-recipients of the gene live significantly longer. Similar work has been done on a type of worm called a nematode. By causing mutations in a single gene that controls antioxidant production in the worm, scientists have extended its lifespan from twenty-five to approximately forty days.

In humans, there appear to be about two hundred genes that control important features of aging. If we tinker successfully with some of these genes, we may find new ways to strengthen our immune function, expand our antioxidant protection, and control the process of neurological decline that leads directly to diseases of aging such as Parkinson's and Alzheimer's. And the odds of achieving some striking successes on the gene front are certainly being fortified daily by the Human Genome Project: Researchers, funded by the National Institutes of Health, are in the process of identifying the exact location of every human gene. Scheduled completion is in the year 2005.

PUSHING THE PLATE ASIDE

A less interventional (but in some ways more unpleasant) path to long life would appear to be drastic self-restraint. Ever since 1935, scientists have been showing—first with rats and later with worms, fish, mice, spiders, fleas, guppies, and snails—that rigorous caloric restriction will greatly extend life span, often by 40 to 50 percent. This restriction, of course, does not involve nutritional deprivation. The animals are fed less, often around one-third of what they would normally eat, but the food is carefully selected for optimal nutritional value, and, in some cases, nutritional supplements are added to the package.

Will this work in humans? To some extent, probably yes. In the late 1980s researchers decided to move up the mammalian tree and find something closer to us. They chose rhesus monkeys and squirrel monkeys, which have average life expectancies of forty and twenty years, respectively. Although the experiment has not been under way long enough to measure changes in life span, the researchers soon found that the thinner and fitter monkeys, which caloric restriction produced, were also healthier monkeys. Unlike well-fed monkeys (and humans), their blood sugar metabolism remained healthy. They had lower levels of blood sugar and remained sensitive to the action of insulin, thus cutting down the probability of diabetes and heart disease, preeminent diseases of aging. Their immune systems also functioned at a higher level than their well-fed brethren.

It's anyone's guess why caloric restriction works, but it appears likely that by reducing the sum total of metabolic events in the body, one actually lowers the body temperature, lowers the rate of free radical reactions, and slows the rate of aging.

Most scientists now think that caloric restriction would be a valid method of extending the life span, if anyone wanted to do it. But the truth is the pool of candidates who are willing to go hungry for the rest of their lives is an extremely limited one.

GOING ON FOREVER?

These approaches to longevity are certainly diversely promising, but they have a limitation. They extend life. But they do no more than that. What if it were possible to not only slow and temporarily reverse aging but actually end it? Some reputable and well-credentialed scientists are speculating that this treasured dream of utopians, science fiction writers, and other visionaries is not only possible but imminent. If they've got it right, then, in as little as a decade or less, the aging process may simply *stop*.

If, at this stage of medical development, we can't even theoretically expect to live forever, it's principally because the one hundred trillion cells in our bodies have a life span limitation. Very simply, our cells can divide only so many times before they begin to age and die—and since the cells in our bodies must divide to reproduce themselves, this certainly puts us in a bind.

You see, the cells in your body get old and senescent— damaged as it were by hard use. Some of them fade quite quickly. Your skin cells might last a few days, the cells in your intestine some weeks, muscle cells a few months. Once they start wearing out, however, your cells have an answer: they simply clone themselves. They produce a daughter cell that's young and viable. Initally it grows on the side of the original cell like a little bud and then it detaches itself. When the old cell dies you haven't lost much. After all, it hatched a replacement.

This replacement cell is not yet specialized. It needs to be taught its role in the body, and this is where hormones come into play. It is under their stimulation and control that the body's new cells mature. Without growth hormone and testosterone, for instance, new cells in your biceps will have a difficult time forming new muscle fiber.

But, of course, for the hormones to perform their magic, they must have the cells to work with, and we now know that though our cells reproduce themselves quite effectively, they can do so only a limited number of times. This catch-22 is why even the luckiest, smartest, best-preserved human being will begin to crack up and disintergrate somewhere between 110 and 120. Too many of his or her cells have died and are dying by then, and too many vital organ systems are being compromised and weakened.

Why do our cells die? Why do they age? It might be for a whole host of reasons, but, in truth, science has discovered only one. The reason why our cells cannot continue dividing eternally like a single-celled amoeba—why, after a finite number of divisions, even the most freshly created cell shows signs of age as soon as its born—is that the end segments of DNA on the chromosomes in each and every one of our cells is capped with something called a telomere. You can visualize these telomeres as being like beads or counters. Typically, at birth, there are approximately 5,000 telemores at the end of each chromosome in an average cell. Every time this average cell divides and replaces itself, one telomere is lopped off in the replacement cell. At first, this has little significance, but, as the years pass and one by one these little top pieces are snapped off, your cellular clock begins to wind down. Eventually, the cell reaches a point at which its functioning is compromised.

It turns out that for a number of reasons—I shall cite two—the telomeres that form the tips of each of your cell's chromosomes are—even though expendable—also essential.

First, the telomere protects the end of the chromosome from damage or faulty recombination. You have ninety-two chromosomes in each of your cells; this is your genetic "library," the coded information that instructs your body in its duties, as well as making you you. Your body is so efficient about controlling you through the genetic code that this code is accurately repeated in every one of your hundred trillion cells. Now, without the telomere capping its tips, it appears that a chromosome may break apart and fuse with another chromosome. This can result in the destruction or disorganization of genetic information. If such an event occurs, the cell cannot survive.

Second, the telomere acts as a buffer, sacrificing a piece of itself when the cell divides and recopies its chromosomes. Without the telomere, a piece of the crucial DNA, on top of which the telomere sits, would be lost. The body does not tolerate the risk or the reality of such errors, and, so, when the telomere comes to an end, the cell is identified as containing damaged DNA, and it receives a message to self-destruct. And, with great reliability, our cells do just that. They die at different rates and in different corners of our anatomy depending upon their frequency of cell division and the number of telomeres that they had to start with. But eventually, the cells of essential organs—your liver, for instance—begin to age and die. When sufficient liver cells are lost, the liver dies, and when the liver dies, the person dies. And a similar litany could be recited for the heart, the kidneys, and the lungs.

This sounds pretty final, doesn't it? Telomeres shorten, cells die, organ dies, you die. Strangely enough, for something that occurs so predictably, this process may not be final or inevitable at all. We now know that the body has the ability to rebuild telomeres. Every cell in our body possesses a gene that when activated produces an enzyme called telomerase. Its sole purpose is the recreation—the relengthening—of the telomeres.

Because this enzyme can be called into existence, some of our cells—namely cancer cells—have the ability to kill us. Cancer cells have solved the trick of activating the gene for telomerase. It's their final trick. A cancer cell has already performed the difficult task of taking the damaged DNA that makes it what it is past the various cellular checkpoints that are supposed to catch and destroy inappropriate genetic variations. Now it can begin dividing, passing on its outlaw "mentality" to its cellular children. But doing that isn't enough. Such a cell is merely regarded as pre-cancerous. It has the will to carry out a predatory path of conquest but, by and large, not the ability. Most such cells die because, in the course of their rapid division and multiplication, they eventually hit the telomere limit. And like any other cell, once it runs out of telomeres, a potential cancer cell is cooked. Time's up, game's over.

However, a very small number of these pre-cancer cells—by one estimate, approximately one in three million—find out how to activate the gene for telomerase. From that point on they continually release the telomerase enzyme and thereby become capable of an infinite number of cell divisions. This occurs quite rapidly. A cancer cell doesn't wait until it gets old and near its end to reproduce, as normal cells do; it divides more or less immediately. Growth, therefore, is exponential. One cell becomes two, two become four, four become eight, and so on. And you, unless your immune system succeeds in destroying this little Hitler, have the beginnings of a cancer.

I suppose it's curious that the one part of us we don't wish to see prosper—malignant cells—has solved the puzzle of immortality to its own satisfaction. If it wasn't that cancers eventually kill us, they would be immortal. They are not, however, quite alone. Another type of cell in the human body—sperm in the male, egg or ova in the female—show no signs of aging. Their immortality is quite necessary since they become the next generation and then the next generation after that, and so on. The immortality of the species is preserved by the immortality of the cells that continue it and have been doing so for countless thousands of years. These cells also rely on telomerase to protect them from the fatal effects of telomere shortening.

The rest of our body has no share in this exemption from aging. And yet, it appears highly probable that it will be within our power to change that. Actually, since the gene for activating telomerase exists in every cell, it is hard to imagine that the telomere clock won't eventually be reset by biological engineering. Michael Fossel, Ph.D., M.D., in a new book called *Reversing Human Aging*, has proposed several methods by which the trick may be accomplished. Moreover, as he points out, control over the telomeres is a two-way street. If we can induce the release of telomerase in the body's cells, we can presumably also inhibit telomerase thereby shutting down cancers.

Research on both these fronts is going on right now. Scientists at the Geron Corporation in California were able to isolate the first examples of telomerase inhibitors in 1994. Initial results show them to be effective against lab specimens of ovarian cancer cells. Further research is being done, including work at Memorial Sloan-Kettering on animals with cancers.

Research is also being done on telomerase inducers at the University of Texas Southwestern Medical Center and at Cold Spring Harbor Laboratory. What we would need to regrow our telomeres is a substance that "turns on" the telomerase gene in each and every one of our cells. One of the places where they'll certainly be looking for telomerase inducers is in the drug libraries of the large pharmaceutical firms which contain the formulas of hundreds of thousands of drugs that have never come to market.

At first glance, there would seem to be an inherent contradiction in both suppressing telomerase to kill cancers and inducing it to extend life. Actually, there shouldn't be a conflict. A chemical inducer of telomerase sets in motion a one-time process. When administered a telomerase inducer will cause our cells to produce telomerase. Once administration is halted, however, telomerase production will stop since our cells are designed to actively suppress telomerase genes. But during the period of administration, the telomeres will have been able to grow. After a certain number of years to will be necessary to administer the inducer yet again so as to grow the telomeres once more.

In the case of cancer, telomerase is continually produced. A telomerase inhibitor, therefore, will not shorten the length of the telomeres in the healthy cells of our bodies, nor, indeed, will it shorten cancer cell telomeres. It will, however, stop the cancer from releasing further telomerase. The cancer's rate of cell division is so fast that it will soon exhaust its telomeres and perish.

It may well be that when telomere therapy is perfected, a telomerase inducer will always be preceded or followed by a telomerase inhibitor in order to kill any cancer cells in the body.

If, indeed, we succeed in inducing the release of telomerase into our cells, the changes will be interesting and profound. Although we won't necessarily be able to repair serious damage that has already been done to our bodies, we will be working with a rejuvenated crop of cells. The health of our organs will improve, our skins will thicken if we're already old, and, at a cellular level, we will cease to grow old. We will essentially stop aging—with some improvements—at whatever age we've already reached.

Could this really be the human future?

WHAT ARE WE ABOUT TO DO?

Aging is no disease, aging is just nature. Right? There is certainly sound biological logic in making that argument. And yet . . . you and I have noticed that human beings treat aging as a disease. They do everything in their power to control it, slow it, and reverse it when they can.

We're about to vastly extend quality life with hormone replacement. Genetic engineering may well prove to be of equal benefit. And waiting in the wings is telomeric engineering. If that comes to pass, our very understanding of human life will be altered radically. A human being who can live a vital, energetic life for two hundred years is an unknown quantity. How will he combine the wisdom of his—or her—experience with the forcefulness of relative metabolic youth? We may, indeed, be on the verge of creating a new type of human being. Perhaps a better type. Certainly a different type.

We will have to adapt to our new knowledge and potentiality. Civilization will have to adapt, too. Retiring at sixty-five is not going to make much sense if that isn't even going to be the halfway point in the span of a normal, active life. Personally, I think these complexities are a welcome alternative to the simplicity of dying. We are creative beings, and if we must create ourselves anew under novel conditions, it will not be beyond our power. We will do it because we must—and if our vastly extended lives expose us to new truths seen under the clear, crisp light of wider horizons, then, who knows, perhaps the truth will make us free.

Appendices

Thyroid

I think we've made it evident in writing this book that our purpose is not only to show you how to live longer but to live younger with all your functional capacities intact and your zest for life burning steady. However, it can be hard to do this if your thyroid gland has turned the temperature down.

You'll probably recall from Chapter Two that the thyroid is an important part of your endocrine system. It maintains your body's temperature and controls the production of energy in your cells. If your thyroid malfunctioned too wildly, you'd simply die. Some people do, you know.

The thyroid hormones can't, I think, be regarded as pro-longevity hormones, which is why I've relegated this material to an appendix, but they do affect how your other hormones work. If your thyroid is out of kilter, then the energy factory in every cell in your body is functioning less efficently. You're healing less efficently, constructing new protein less efficently, and making use of your other endocrine hormones—the pro-longevity hormones discussed in this book—very poorly.

Let's consider what can go wrong with your thyroid, because if you're doing everything else right and you're still not feeling good, there's a very good chance that abnormally high or low thyroid function is the culprit. Up to 20 percent of people over sixty years old—women more commonly than men—have thyroid problems. An appallingly high percentage are undiagnosed.

HIGH OR LOW

Thyroid hormones are produced in the thyroid gland, in the front of the neck, just under the Adam's apple. The pituitary gland controls production by its secretion of thyroid stimulating hormone (TSH), which increases or decreases according to perceived need.

Thyroid hormone can become excessive because of a tumor on the thyroid or pituitary glands or because of an antibody inbalance. When thyroid hormone is abnormally high, nervousness results with excess sweating, tremors, weakness, weight loss, and sometimes a bulging of the eyes. In older people, this condition, known as thyrotoxicosis, can even cause heart failure.

The more common thyroid disorder, however, is a deficiency. This can be caused by an allergic reaction, really a form of auto-immune disease. Viral infections can also destroy thyroid function. But, in many cases, thyroid activity declines to abnormally low levels without any obvious cause except advancing age.

Low thyroid—hypothyroidism—causes sluggishness and low energy. Body temperature goes down, weight gain is common, fluid retention occurs, and cholesterol rises. Generally, the victim of this condition exists in a state of chronic fatigue, and, in extreme cases, the outcome can be coma and death.

In the majority of cases, such disorders are relatively easy to diagnose using common laboratory blood tests of thyroid hormone and TSH levels. If such a deficiency is measured, a doctor will prescribe thyroid hormone tablets taken by mouth. I usually prefer natural, Armour brand desiccated thyroid rather than the synthetic varieties for reasons that I'll explain shortly.

WHAT IF YOUR TESTS ARE NORMAL?

Unfortunately, it's quite possible to get back normal laboratory tests and still have low body temperature causing chronic fatigue. This is functional hypothyroidism. The problem is that a normal amount of thyroid hormone is being released into the circulation, but the hormone is not having its full effect at the cellular level.

To explain this we need to look at the various thyroid hormones. Thyroid hormone is made in the body from an amino acid called tyrosine, which is obtained from dietary protein. On the most common form of thyroid hormone, there are four sites that bind to four iodine molecules, and it is therefore called tetraiodothyronine, or T_4 for short.

Another form of thyroid hormone, which is ten times as potent as T_4, has only three iodine molecules and is called T_3. Although the thyroid gland produces three times as much T_4 as T_3, the liver and other tissues in the body then convert T_4 into T_3 for maximum effectiveness at the cellular level.

We have only recently understood that there is also a third kind of thyroid hormone, really an anti-thyroid hormone. It is part of the body's mechanism for conserving energy. Normal thyroid hormone helps us to utilize energy. Under certain circumstances, however—famine and fasting are the most outstanding examples—the body wants to conserve energy, and it does so by lowering body temperature, lowering energy production, and, generally speaking, slowing us down. It does this by converting T_4 not to T_3 but to reverse T_3, or rT_3. A mirror image of true T_3, rT_3 has an the empty iodine receptor on the reverse side, which binds tightly to thyroid receptors within cells. It thus blocks the action of normal T_3 by denying it landing zones.

The effect produced is somewhat similar to hibernation, and clearly during a famine this decreased energy consumption might be precisely what allows you to stay alive. Highly efficient varieties of this famine response seem to be what makes it so difficult for some people to lose weight. Many people have a hereditary tendency toward prolonged rT_3 production, which dieting activates. Lower energy production partly cancels out the effect of lessened caloric intake, and this low metabolic rate may continue for some time even after the diet is over, hastening weight regain.

Routine laboratory tests will not detect this abnormal ratio of rT_3 to T_3, although some very expensive tests, which have recently been developed, will do so. A much easier test, which costs nothing, is to measure body temperature several times daily with an accurate clinical thermometer. If the average body temperature is consistently below 98 degrees Fahrenheit, inappropriate conversion of T_4 to rT_3 may be the cause. See the box on the following page.

How to Test Yourself for Thyroid Function

Obtain an accurate clinical thermometer made from glass with a silver mercury column inside. Electrical, digital, and color-stripe thermometers are not accurate enough for this purpose. Take your temperature several times—during the part of the day when you are active—each day. Wait for at least three hours after you are out of bed in the morning before you take the first reading and take an additional two readings at least three hours apart. Hold the thermometer in your mouth, under your tongue, for at least five minutes. Keep your mouth completely closed while the thermometer is inserted. Do not eat or drink anything for at least twenty minutes prior to taking your temperature. You want the inside of the your mouth to reflect your core body temperature, not what you recently put into it.

Write down each reading to the nearest tenth of a degree. Women should not do this during the three days prior to or during their menstrual cycle because the temperature is often higher then. Also, your readings should not be done during an acute illness or on days when you are unusually inactive.

Average the three readings for each day (add the three readings together and divide by three). Do this on seven different days. They do not have to be consecutive days.

If the average of the three readings for five or more of the seven days is below 97.8 degrees Fahrenheit, your metabolism is slower than normal and you might have either an absolute deficiency of thyroid hormone or you may be producing too much rT_3 relataive to T_3. Temperatuares from 97.9 to 98.2 degrees may be normal for some people. For other people, temperatures in that range may indicate a thyroid problem. Additional laboratory testing available from a doctor's office can help to make a more accurate diagnosis.

If repeated measurements show that your body temperature is consistently low and the usual lab tests are normal, you should probably move on to those expensive lab tests I mentioned so that your doctor can determine your precise levels of T_3 and rT_3. In a person without an rT_3 problem, the ratio of T_3 to rT_3 should be higher than ten-to-one. Therefore, if your level is lower than that and your body temperature is consistently low, there's an excellent probability that you've found your problem.

Just as most of the pro-longevity hormones decrease with age, it now appears that the conversion of T_4 to rT_3 increases with age, blocking normal thyroid activity in some people. Major stress, such as that resulting from surgery, clinical depression, serious infection, or severe psychological stress factors can also trigger the increased production of rT_3. The condition can become permanent, in which case the body does not return to its normal ratios after the precipitating stress has passed. The problem is best dealt with by taking doses of pure, time-release T_3 by mouth. Slowly increasing doses can often reset the body's thyroid thermostat. Remember that this full program must be prescribed and supervised by a knowledgeable physician. Self-tinkering with ones own thyroid gland would be exceptionally foolish. After a month or so of treatment, the T_3 is slowly tapered and stopped. If body temperature remains normal, it indicates that normal thyroid regulatory mechanisms have been restored.

In dosing with timed-release T_3, begin with 7.5 micrograms (mcg) every twelve hours. Increase the dose by 7.5 mcg after each two days of therapy. Body temperature should be monitored several times each day and averaged until the average temperature for most days is above 98.4 degrees Fahrenheit. Fluctuations from 98.2 to 98.6 are acceptable.

Never exceed 90 mcg of timed-release T_3 in a twelve-hour period. If an increased dose causes you to feel worse, reduce to the next lowest level. If you were on another thyroid medication prior to starting this therapy, your doctor should discontinue it while you're taking timed-release T_3.
Unfortunately, the number of physicians who are currently familar with this approach to thyroid is quite small, but if you suffer from this problem you will have no choice but to find one. You might want to contact the American College for the Advancement of Medicine (ACAM) at 714-583-7666 for a reference. To get pure time-release T_3 you will need to have a prescription filled by a specialized compounding pharmacy.

The one I use is Wellness Pharmacy in Birmingham, AL, at 800-227-2627.

In some cases, of course, the problem is not corrected by treatment with pure time-release T_3, or the real problem is not an overabundance of rT_3 but a more common type of thyroid problem, such as an inability of the thyroid to produce enough hormone. In such situations, the best answer is usually long-term, if not lifetime, treatment with thyroid hormone. My recommendation is the natural Armour thyroid tablets, which contain both T_3 and T_4. The more commonly prescribed synthetic T_4 (currently the most common brand used is called Synthroid) is pure T_4. If the body's conversion of T_4 to T_3 is not adequate, which is sometimes the case, a combination of the two hormones as found in Armour thyroid seem more practical. For some reason most doctors still only prescribe the far less active synthetic T_4, and they rarely measure the T_3/rT_3 ratio.

Thyroid problems—as this short introduction may already have convinced you—are an intensely complex area of medicine. But if you do have an over or under-active thyroid, you never will feel physically well until the problem is fixed. An active energy-consuming creature such as you are can never feel right with a broken thermostat.

Chelation and ACAM

The American College of Advancement in Medicine (ACAM) was founded chiefly as an organization representing doctors who believed in a controversial treatment known as chelation therapy. The treatment is still controversial, but, in my opinion, extremely beneficial. Chelation was developed in the 1940s as a treatment for lead poisoning. It is still (no controversy there) the standard treatment for that problem.

Chelation involves the intravenous administration into the body (generally over a three hour period) of a chemical called EDTA (ethylene diamine tetra acetic acid). EDTA binds heavy metals such as lead, copper, cadmium (and, to a lesser extent, iron) to it, and these metals are then removed from the body through the normal process of excretion.

The health benefits of removing excess quantities of heavy metals from the body are considerable. Dr. Claire Patterson of the California Institute of Technology has estimated that the average modern person is struggling under a body burden of lead that is 1,000 times greater than that of the average person in the pre-modern era.

The main reason, however, that I advise my patients who are middle-aged or older to consider being chelated is that there is very considerable evidence (about which I once wrote a book called *Bypassing Bypass*) that chelation therapy can help restore healthy arteries and reverse the progress of cardiovascular disease.

This is not the place to discuss the reasons why chelation is assumed to work, nor to explain why it remains a subject of controversy. There is reason to hope that an impartial, double-blinded investigation of the therapy will be conducted within the next few years. Hopefully, the results will be unambiguous.

Meanwhile, I would like to recommend ACAM to you as a source of information and referrals. Over the years, ACAM has evolved into an organization which represents many hundreds of innovative physicians. A significant number of them have experience with the pro-longevity hormones. ACAM will be able to provide you with a current directory of their physicians, and they may be able to guide you in your search for a doctor who is competent in this area. Their address is:

American College of Advancement in Medicine
23121 Verdugo Dr., Suite 204
Laguna Hills, CA 92653
(714) 583-7666
Fax (714) 455-9679

Of course, the listing of a physician's name in the ACAM directory does not indicate endorsement by the authors of this book. Not all physicians are equally qualified, and their treatment programs will naturally vary. We do hope, however, that the information in this book will help you in finding a doctor with whom you feel comfortable and in whom you have confidence.

Compounding and Anti-Aging Pharmacies

These are pharmacies that your doctor can contact. We don't endorse these particular businesses, but we have noticed that they are often reliable sources for some of the anti-aging hormones.

ApotheCure, Inc.
13720 Midway Rd., Ste. 109
Dallas, TX 75244
(800) 969-6601

Bajamar Women's HealthCare Pharmacy
9609 Dielman Rock Island
St. Louis, MO 63132
314-997-3414

California Pharmacy and Compounding Center, Inc.
307 Placentia Ave., #0102
Newport Beach, CA 92663
714-642-8057

College Pharmacy
833 N. Tejon
Colorado Springs, CO 80903
(800) 888-9358

Homelink Pharmacy
2650 Elm Ave., Ste. 104
Long Beach, CA 90806
310-988-0260
(800) 272-4767

Medical Center Pharmacy
10721 Main St.
Fairfax, VA 22030
703-273-7311

Wellness Health and Pharmaceuticals, Inc.
2800 South 18th St.
Birmingham, AL 35209
(800) 227-2627

Women's International Pharmacy
5708 Monona Drive
Madison, WI 53716
608-221-7800
Fax 608-221-7819
also:
13925 Meeker Blvd., Suite #13
Sun City West, AZ 85375
602-214-7700
Fax 602-214-7708

References

Chapter One: The Promise of Longevity

1. Rudman, D., et al. "Effects of human growth hormone in men over 60 years old," *The New England Journal of Medicine*, 1990; 323: 1–6.

Chapter Three: Human Growth Hormone

1. Op. cit. Rudman et al.

Chapter Four: The Body of Evidence

1. Kelley, K. W., et al. "GH3 pituitary adenoma cells can reverse thymic aging in rats," *Proceedings of the National Academy of Science*, 1986; 83: 5663–5667.
2. Monroe, W. E., et al. "Effect of growth hormone on the adult canine thymus," *Thymus*, 1987; 9: 173–187.
3. Khansari, D. N., and Gustad, T. "Effects of long-term, low-dose growth hormone therapy on immune function and life expectancy of mice," *Mechanisms of Aging and Development*, 1991; 57: 87–100.
4. Crist, D. M., et al. "Exogenous growth hormone treatment alters body composition and increases natural killer cell activity in women with impaired endogenous growth hormone secretion," *Metabolism*, 1987; 36 (12): 1115–1117.
5. Fabris, N., et al. "Recovery of age-related decline of thymic endocrine activity and PHA response by llysin-arginine combination," *International Journal of Immunopharmacology*, 1986; 8: 677–685.
6. Aroonsakul, C. "Reduced Growth Hormone in Alzheimer's Disease," *Journal of Advancement in Medicine*, 1995; 8 (3): 206–208.
7. Clemmesen, B., et al. "Human growth hormone and growth hormone releasing hormone: a double-masked, placebo-controlled study of their effects on bone metabolism in elderly women," *Osteoporosis International*, 1993; 3: 330–336.
8. Personal communication from Edmund Chein, M.D.
9. Cittadini, A., et al. "Impaired cardiac performance in hGH-deficient adults and its improvement after hGH replacement," *American Journal of Physiology*, 1994; 267 (*Endocrinol. Metab.* 30): E219–E225.

10. Personal communication from David R. Clemmons, M.D., at the University of North Carolina School of Medicine.

11. Papadikis, M. A., et al. "Growth hormone replacement in healthy older men improves body composition but not functional ability," *Annals of Internal Medicine*, 1996; 124 (8): 708–716.

Chapter Five: Growth Hormone

1. Fradkin, J. E., et al. "Risk of leukemia after treatment with pituitary growth hormone," *Journal of the American Medical Association*, 1993; 270: 2829–2832.

2. Ogilvy-Stuart, A.L., et al. "Growth hormonal and tumor recurrence," *British Medical Journal*, 1992; 304: 1601–1605.

Chapter Six: DHEA

1. Morales, A. J., et al. "Effects of replacement dose of dehydroepiandrosterone in men and women of advancing age," *Journal of Clinical Endocrinology and Metabolism*, 1994; 78 (6): 1360–1367.

2. Barrett-Connor, E., et al. "A prospective study of dehydroepiandrosterone sulfate, mortality and cardiovascular disease," *The New England Journal of Medicine*, 1986; 315 (24): 1519–1524.

3. Gordon, G. B., et al. "Reduction of atherosclerosis by administration of dehydroepinandrosterone," *Journal of Clinical Investigation*, 1988; 82: 712–720.

4. Eich, D. M., et al. "Inhibition of accelerated coronary atherosclerosis with dehydroepiandrosterone in the heterotopic rabbit model of cardiac transplanation," *Circulation*, 1993; 87 (1): 261–269.

5. Personal communication from Raymond Daynes, Ph.D. at the University of Arizonia.

6. Ben-Nathan, D., et al. "Dehyroepinadrosterone protects mice inoculated with West Nile virus and exposed to cold stress," *Journal of Medical Virology*, 1992; 38 (3): 159–166.

7. Bulbrook, R. D. "Relations between urinary androgen and corticoid excretion and subsequent breast cancer," *Lancet*, 1971; v.ii: 395–398.

8. Rudman, D., et al. "Plasma dehydroepiandrosterone sulfate in nursing home men," *Journal of the American Geriatrics Society*, 1990; 38(4): 421–427.

Chapter Seven: The Melatonin Magical Mystery Tour

1. Reiter, R. J. "Oxidative Processes and Antioxidative Defense Mechanisms in the Aging Brain," *FASEB Journal*, 1995; 9 (7): 526–33.

2. Lerner, A. B., *Journal of the American Chemical Society*, 1958.

3. Pierpaoli, W., et al. "Pineal grafting and melatonin induce immunocompetence in nude (athymic) mice," *International Journal of Neuroscience*, 1993; 68: 123–131.

4. Pierpaoli, W., et al. "The pineal control of aging. The effects of melatonin and pineal grafting on the survival of older mice," *Annals of the New York Academy of Sciences*, 1991; 621: 291–313.

5. Lesnikov, V. A., and Pierpaoli, W. "Pineal cross-transplantation (old-to-young and vice versa) as evidence for an endogenous 'aging clock,'" *Annals of the New York Academy of Sciences*, 1994; 719: 456–60.

6. Virginia Utermohlen, unpublished study, Cornell University.

7. Maestroni, G. J., et al. "Pineal melatonin, its fundamentnal immunoregula-

tory role in aging and cancer," *Annals of the New York Academy of Sciences*, 1988; 521: 140–148.

8. Ben-Nathan, D., et al. "Protective effects of melatonin in mice infected with encephalitis virus," *Archives of Virology*, 1995; 140: 223–230.

9. Maestroni, G. J. "T-helper-2 lympocytes as peripheral target of melatonin signaling," *Journal of Pineal Research*, 1995; 18: 84-89.

10. Tamarkin, L., et al. "Melatonin inhibition and pinealectomy enhancement of 7,12-Dimethylbenz( )anthracene-induced mammary tumors in the rat," *Cancer Research*, 1981; 41: 4432–4436.

11. Blask, D. E., and Hill, S. M. "Effects of melatonin on cancer: studies on MCF-7 human breast cancer cells in culture," *Journal of Neural Transmission*, 1986; 21: 433–449.

12. Cohen, M., et al. "Role of pineal gland in etiiology and treatment of breast cancer," *Lancet*, 1978: 814–816.

13. Wilson, S. T., et al. "Melatonin augments the sensitivity of MCF-7 human breast cancer cells to tamoxifen in vitro," *Journal of Clinical Endocrinology and Metabolism*, 1992; 75 (2): 669–670.

14. Lissoni, P., and Barni, S. *British Journal of Cancer*, 1995; 71: 001–003.

15. Lissoni, P., et al. "A randomized study with subcutaneous low-dose inter-leukin 2 alone vs interleukin 2 plus the pineal neurohormone melatonin in advanced solid meoplasms other than renal cancer and melanoma," *British Journal of Cancer*, 1994; 69: 196–199.

16. Lissoni, P., et al. "A randomized study of immunotherapy with low-dose subcutaneous interleukin-2 plus melatonin vs chemotherapy with cisplatin and etoposide as first-line therapy for advanced non-small cell lung cancer," *Tumori*, 1994; 80: 464–467.

Chapter Eight: Melatonin: Sleep King

1. Steinberg, R., and Soyka, M. "Problems in long-term benzodiazepine treat-ment," *Schweizerische Rundschaufur Medizin Praxis*, 1989; 78: 784–787.

2. Lieberman, H. R., et al. "Effects of melatonin on human mood and perfor-mance," *Brain Research*, 1984; 323: 201–207.

Chapter Nine: Estrogen

1. Ettinger, B., et al. "Reduced mortality associated with long-term post-menopausal estrogen therapy," *Obstetrics and Gynecology*, 1996; 87: 6–12.

2. Prior, J. C. "Progesterone as a bone-trophic hormone," *Endocrine Reviews*, 1990; 11 (2): 386–398.

3. Hammond, C. B., et al. "Effects of long-term estrogen replacement therapy," *American Journal of Obstetrics and Gynecology*, 1979; 133: 525–536.

4. Cauley, J. A. "Estrogen replacement therapy & fractures in older women," *Annals of Internal Medicine*, 1995; 122 (1): 9–16.

5. Henderson, V. W., et al. "Estrogen replacement therapy in older women. Comparisions between Alzheimer's disease cases and nondemented control sub-jects," *Archives of Neurology*, 1994; 51 (9): 896–900.

6. Paganini-Hill, A., and Henderson, V. W. "Estrogen deficiency and risk of Alzheimer's disease in women," *American Journal of Epidemiology*, 1994; 140 (3): 256–261.

7. Robinson, D., et al. "Estrogen replacement therapy and memory in older women," *Journal of the American Geriatrics Society*, 1994; 42 (9): 919–922.

8. Follingstad, A. H., "Estriol, the forgotten estrogen," *Journal of the American Medical Association*, 1978; 239: 29–30.

9. "Effects of estrogen or estrogen/progestin regimens on heart disease risk factors in postmenopausal women. The Postmenopausal Estrogen/Progestin Interventions (PEPI) Trial," *Journal of the American Medical Association*, 1995; 273 (3): 199–208.

10. Presentation by Dr. Angela Bowen at annual meeting of the North American Menopause Society, November, 1995.

11. Sherwin, B. B. "A comparative analysis of the role of androgen in human male and female sexual behavior: behavioral specificity, critical thresholds, and sensitivity," *Psychobiology*, 1988; 16: 416–425.

See also: Young, R. L., et al. "Comparision of estrogen plus androgen and estrogen on libido and sexual satisfaction in recently oophorectomized women," *Abstracts of North American Menopause Society*, Montreal, September 1991, p.103.

12. Newcomb, P. A., and Storer, B. E. "Postmenopausal hormone use and risk of large-bowel cancer," *Journal of the National Cancer Institute*, 1995; 87: 1067–1071.

Chapter Ten: Testosterone

1. Hoberman, J. M., and Yesalis, C. E. "The History of Synthetic Testosterone," *Scientific American*, February 1995.

2. Phillips, G. B., et al. "The association of hypotestosteronemia with coronary artery disease in men," *Arteriosclerosis and Thrombosis*, 1994; 14 (5): 701–706.

3. Marin, P., et al. "The effects of testosterone treatment on body composition and metabolism in middle-aged obese men," *International Journal of Obesity*, 1992; 16: 991–997.

4. Tenover, J. S. "Effects of testosterone supplementation in the aging male," *Journal of Clinical Endocrinology and Metabolism*, 1992; 75 (4): 1092–1098.

5. Lichtenstein, M. J. "Sex hormones, insulin, lipids, and prevalent ischemic heart disease," *American Journal of Epidemiology*, 1987; 126 (4): 647–657.

Index

About the Authors

Elmer M. Cranton, M.D., graduated from Harvard Medical School in 1964. He currently practices chelation therapy, hyperbaric oxygen therapy, general and preventive medicine at the Mount Rogers Clinic, Trout Dale, Virginia—high in the beautiful Blue Ridge Mountains. He also has a satellite clinic in Yelm, Washington. Dr. Cranton is a diplomate of both the American Board of Family Practice and the American Board of Chelation Therapy. He is Past President of the Smyth County Medical Society, Past President of the American Holistic Medical Association, Past President of the American College for Advancement in Medicine, and he has served as Chief-of-Staff at the U.S. Public Health Service hospital.

Elmer M. Cranton, M.D.
Mount Rogers Clinic
P.O. Box 44—799 Ripshin Road
Trout Dale, VA 24378-0044
(540) 677-3631
FAX: (540) 677-3843

Elmer M. Cranton, M.D.
Mount Ranier Clinic
503 First Street South, Suite 1
P. O. Box 7510
Yelm, WA 98597-7510
(800) 337-9918 or (360) 458-1061
FAX: (360) 458-1661

William Fryer graduated from Georgetown University, was a senior editor at a New York publishing house, and for the past ten years has written in the health and medical fields. He was assistant editor of *Dr. Atkins' Health Revelations*, a national newsletter, and has co-authored five books, the most recent being *Unmasking PMS*.